How Queer!

How Queer!

Personal narratives from bisexual, pansexual, polysexual, sexually-fluid, and other non-monosexual perspectives

Compiled by Faith Beauchemin

On Our Own Authority! Publishing.
Atlanta, Georgia

How Queer! –
Personal narratives from bisexual, pansexual, polysexual, sexually-fluid, and other non-monosexual perspectives.

Compiled and introduced by Faith Anne Beauchemin.

Copyright © 2016

On Our Own Authority! Publishing.
Atlanta, Georgia.

All rights reserved. This book may not be reproduced in any form by any electronic or mechanical means including photocopying, recording, or information storage and retrieval without permission in writing from the publisher.

ISBN-13: 978-0-9906418-2-7
ISBN-10: 0-9906418-2-1
LCCN: 2015920163

www.oooabooks.org
oooabooks@gmail.com

Cover art by Julia Simoniello

CONTENTS

Acknowledgements	7
Glossary	9
Part One: Introduction	
A Note on the Title	14
Preface	15
"Placing the Personal Narrative in Context," an introduction by Faith Beauchemin	18
Part Two: Narratives	
"The Invisible B," by Faith Beauchemin	25
"Not Straight … Or Anything Else For That Matter," by Hugh Goldring	29
"Flying In the Face Of Everything," by Kierstyn King	37
"(Un)Seen," by J	41
"What You See Isn't What You Get," by Lucas	44
"I Could Pick A Side … But I Won't," by Liam H. Smith	47
"Call The Doctor," by M	50
"Landmines," by Marie	54
"Life, Take 2," by Courgette	59
"I Am More Than My Sexual Orientation," by Beth Desmontagnes	62

"To Be Or Not To Be," by Danielle Hamilton	65
"It Shouldn't Have To Be a Secret," by Grace Carrol	67
"So Tell Me About Your Childhood: How Therapy Saved My Sexuality and Sense Of Self," by Johnnie Stevens	69
"Mother Of Pearl," by Sophie Unruh	74

Part Three: Reflection and Analysis

Bisexuality and Culture	81
Bisexuality in Queer Politics and the Changing American Family	89
A Personal Look At Bisexuality	101
Bisexuality in the "LGBT" Community	108
The Bisexual Community, Allyship, Activism, and Revolutionary Potential	114

Bibliography	125

ACKNOWLEDGMENTS

Writing a book is a team effort. I was astonished to find just how many people were involved in the process, and more, how many people were constantly ready with support, encouragement, and the help I needed. In addition to each and every amazing individual who entrusted me with their essays for this collection, I would like to thank the following people: Andrew Zonneveld and Mettie June, without whose careful and patient editing this book would literally never have been possible. The folks at Homeschoolers Anonymous and Citizen Radio, and the communities associated with each—your willingness to help me plug the project at the outset was vital. Erek, whose unwavering support and faith gave me the necessary motivation to just do the thing. My parents, who would hate everything about this book but always encouraged my dreams of writing when I was young. I did it, Mom and Dad. You may never know about it, but I did it. And all my wonderful middle-of-the-rainbow friends, those who wrote for this book and those who didn't. Your support—knowing you were there, knowing I was not alone—is more important to me than any of you will ever know.

GLOSSARY

This is by no means an exhaustive list, but it briefly summarizes the terms related to gender and sexuality that may be unfamiliar to some readers.

Agender: One who does not have a gender.

Asexual: Not sexually attracted to anyone. May or may not experience romantic attraction.

Bigender: One who identifies as having two genders.

Binary: A system of two opposing options with no choices in between. E.g., you can be heterosexual or homosexual but nothing else; you can be male or female but nothing else.

Bisexual: Attracted to people of more than one gender, though not necessarily all, and not necessarily equally or in a static, unchanging way. This word is frequently used for ease of reference as it is a familiar term to many people; it is not meant imply that a person identifying as bisexual is attracted only to people of binary genders.

Biphobia: An aversion towards, and source of discrimination against,

Glossary

bisexuality and bisexual people. Often based on fear and negative stereotypes.

Cisgender: Identifying with the gender one was assigned at birth. (The prefix "cis" is often used instead of the entire word.)

Cishet: A portmanteau of "cisgender" and "heterosexual." This word is often used as shorthand for a non-queer person.

Genderfluid: One whose gender varies between different points along the spectrum or the binary, or is off the spectrum altogether.

Genderqueer: One whose gender does not fit into the binary.

Heterosexist: Enforcing the assumption that heterosexuality is the only real sexuality. May include the idea that queer relationships are attempting to mimic heterosexual relationships.

Homosexual: Attracted to people of one's own gender.

Heterosexual: Attracted to only one gender that is not one's own.

Monogamy: Having sexual and/or romantic relationships with only one person at a time.

Monosexist: Enforcing the assumption that one can only be attracted to people of one gender; see also *biphobia*.

Monosexual: Attracted to people of only one gender, whether that is one's own gender or a different gender. Includes *heterosexual* and *homosexual*.

Non-Binary: Existing outside the two opposing choices presented in a binarist system. E.g., I am neither heterosexual nor homosexual; I am neither a man nor a woman.

Pansexual: Attracted to people of all genders, though not necessarily equally or in a static way.

Polyamory: Having sexual and/or romantic relationships with more than one person at a time, in an open and honest manner respectful to all partners involved.

Polysexual: Attracted to people of multiple genders, but not necessarily all genders.

Sexually fluid: Attraction varies among more than one gender. May include switching between various labels and identifiers.

Transgender: One whose gender differs from the gender they were assigned at birth. They may identify with non-binary genders or the gender opposite their assigned gender on the binary, and they may choose to pursue hormone and/or surgical treatment or not. (The prefix *trans* or *trans** is often used instead of the entire word).

PART ONE: INTRODUCTION

A NOTE ON THE TITLE

"Dear, dear! How queer everything is today! And yesterday things went on just as usual. I wonder if I've been changed in the night? . . . But if I'm not the same, the next question is, Who in the world am I?"
— *Alice's Adventures in Wonderland*, Lewis Carroll.

"How queer," characters in old literature exclaim or muse upon confronting something unexpected or out of the ordinary. Today, the primary use of the word is in reference to non-heterosexual and/or non-cisgender people. Whether taken as derogatory or as a badge of pride is determined based on the context. However, for people who fall somewhere in the middle of the sexuality spectrum, or outside of the sexuality binary, "queer" retains both meanings. We are, of course, something other than heterosexual; we are regarded as strange, out of the ordinary, odd, and by some, as fantastical as Alice's adventures down the rabbit hole.

"How Queer!" is a bold statement, an exclamation that our identity is indeed something distinctly outside of the cisgender, heterosexual norm, and we are not going to hide it. We insist upon living our own reality. We are not a fantasy, even as we find within ourselves the peculiar seeds of a future that not everyone else is willing to acknowledge.

PREFACE

WHEN I CAME OUT AS BI, I WAS SHOCKED TO DISCOVER just how many people in my circle of acquaintances and friends also identified as bisexual, pansexual, sexually fluid, and otherwise attracted to people of more than one gender. Sexual identity wasn't something we often talked about; many of them would have never said a word to me about it if I hadn't come out directly. I came out in a blogpost, and through that the thought occurred—if I asked my friends to write about their sexuality, what would they say? What similarities would emerge, and what differences? How might all of us telling our stories help others, especially those like us?

If there existed a collection of personal narratives by ordinary people (not academics or professional activists) about their journeys along the non-monosexual spectrum, could it encourage other people who are told constantly by society that their sexuality is nonexistent, fake, or wrong, to celebrate and love themselves? Could it help them to begin to live in hope instead of in hiding?

Although I feared that publishing stories about sexuality would be too reductive, I soon found that no life story is so small that it can be crudely simplified. Like every other form of identity, sexuality is only one part of the whole picture. An understanding of sexuality frequently evolves alongside personal beliefs and values, and sometimes that understanding may be a

Preface

catalyst for disruption in personal life. Each person who contributed to this book is a fully-rounded human being, with their own gender, belief system, values, background, interests and social relationships.

By telling our own stories, we are pushing back against reductive narratives, stereotypes, and a heterosexist, monosexist society. We are not what such a society expects, but we can be pleasantly surprised by looking around at who inhabits our shared community.

It is difficult, if not impossible, to discuss sexuality without concurrently discussing a whole host of other issues. In conversations of gender, family structure, the vast spectrum of political movements, or understanding the ways we might bring about social change, it is important to note that sexuality is necessarily entwined in one way or another with most aspects of discussion, and indeed, our lives. By coming out and taking that one step further toward living authentically, I've learned that my sexuality's existence outside of culturally approved boxes can only enhance my activism and interests in other areas.

I will be the first to admit that I am not good at offering concrete action plans for activism and change. My strengths lie in historical and social analysis, and suggesting potential starting points for a way forward. However I might personally envision a future we should work toward, I believe our ultimate goals must be creatively imagined by our community working together—not by any one person.

This book, therefore, does not contain a grand action plan or map to get us from where we are currently to a liberated future. I have sought purely to present the stories of many different non-monosexual people, alongside reflections and analyses that explore the challenges and opportunities faced by non-monosexual people individually and as a community.

These analyses are limited to an examination of bisexuality in the United States; although some of the narratives presented are from elsewhere (including India, New Zealand, and Canada).

Whether you've been an out and proud bisexual for many decades, or are completely in the closet and unsure of whether or not you'll ever be able to come out, I want this book to give you hope and a sense of community. Many others have made the same journey you are on, each in their own way. Within these pages perhaps you will recognize things long in your past, or

Preface

perhaps you will come up with a potential roadmap for your own future. Whatever the case, may this book bring you comfort, help, and a refreshed vision of a more rainbow world that we can create together.

INTRODUCTION:
Placing The Personal Narrative in Context

"Imagine bisexuality as a space for difficulty, discomfort, and disruption—not as simple disturbance, problems to be solved, or barriers to overcome, but as sites of complexity whose very virtues are contradictions, inconsistencies, and incongruities." — Shiri Eisner[1]

"What new possibilities arise when we learn to cross, to blur, to undermine, or overflow the hierarchical and binary oppositions we have been taught to believe in?" — Jamie Heckert[2]

IN TODAY'S SOCIETY, WE ARE TAUGHT THAT GENDER AND SEXUALITY are only to be allowed one way. Although the existence of LGBT identities are more or less acknowledged (depending on which identity is being discussed), these identities are still not endorsed by mainstream society. Normal people—the people who get to be heroes and have happy endings—are usually white,

---

1 Shiri Eisner, *Bi: Notes for a Bisexual Revolution* (Berkeley, CA: Seal Press, 2013), 113.
2 Jamie Heckert, "Anarchy Without Opposition," in *Queering Anarchism: Addressing and Understanding Power and Desire*, ed. C. B. Daring et al. (Oakland, CA: AK Press, 2012), 50.

cisgender, heterosexual (cishet) people. If you're queer, you are at best a flamboyant best friend, or proof that the hero is an accepting, open minded person. At worst, you may be the vilified victim or perpetrator of violence, but most often you are simply a punch line. The right way to be—the way happy, successful, accepted people are—is cisgender and heterosexual. Anything else is of a lesser caliber, and tearing down binaries is unheard of.

Non-monosexuality is inherently disruptive of gender and sexuality norms. Instead of fitting easily into categories organized by proximity to the approved monogamous, cisgender, and heterosexual standard, we are often transgressive. Our very existence in the middle of or even completely outside of the spectrum raises questions that the straight, monogamous establishment tries to keep tidily swept under the rug.

Is it possible to color outside the lines, to leave well-worn trails and discover that there is more possible in love and sexuality than those in power want us to believe? Whether we gradually knock down wall after wall like dominoes or, having been oppressed too long and too harshly, we simply explode and wash away all barriers at once, every box we transcend leads to other possibilities. Living and loving outside the strictures of "ought to," and "should," and "what someone else approves of" paves the way for greater freedom than we ever foresaw.

In our culture, sexuality comes with a certain set of assumptions. It is expected that a person can only be in love with one other person at a time. It is expected that said monogamous relationships should have a masculine partner and a feminine partner, an assumption that also plagues popular perceptions of queer relationships and enforces heterosexism even in non-heterosexual spaces. It is also expected that a person's sexuality will remain static, singular, and unchanged over time.

Bisexuality and other non-monosexual identities chip away at these expectations, raising question after question, opening up possibility after possibility. If I can be in love with a man or a woman, could I also be in love with a person who is both a man and a woman? What about a genderqueer person, an agender person, or a genderfluid person? To what extent is my gender bound up in my perception of my own sexuality? If I do not have to perform the gender role prescribed for me by a heterosexist narrative, might I more deeply examine what I've always been told my gender is? Perhaps I will realize that I am cis, or perhaps I will find myself somewhere in the category

Introduction

of trans, or perhaps I will find myself outside the gender box altogether. Whatever conclusion I come to, I have more deeply considered what gender is and how it makes up part of my identity, which in turn can only deepen my analysis of my personal relation to the world and this huge question of gender and sexuality.

If I remain bisexual even if I am in a relationship with a person of just one gender, how does that challenge the reign of monogamy? Monogamy claims absolute moral right over sexual relationships; the truest love is that which acknowledges attraction only to the beloved, or so the "correct" romantic narrative attempts to convince us. However, non-monosexuals blow the lid off that whole narrative. If I remain attracted to people of more than one gender while dating a person of only one gender, I must admit that I remain attracted to people other than my partner. Is this fact the death knell to a monogamous relationship? Or can I maintain a healthy monogamous relationship even if I am attracted to others? Will society finally be forced to admit that relationships depend not upon matching a perfect, preformed romantic narrative, but upon the trust, love, and daily work contributed by the partners involved?

And if desire continues to spill over to others, even while in a committed monogamous relationship, might we not then explore the possibilities of polyamory as well? This may take much deeper restructuring of the imagination, although (contrary to popular belief) it is a call to a higher standard of character and behavior in relationships. Polyamory can often involve far greater honesty and much less possessiveness and jealousy than monogamous relationships (especially those monogamous relationships entered into mindlessly just because "that's how relationships work"). Polyamory makes explicit the necessity for relationships to be a meeting of autonomous, fully consenting adults who can be honest with and respectful of each other.

If a bisexual person is in a relationship with two or more people of differing genders, what will happen if they were to want to marry each other? Is it possible that marriage is just another aspect of the stifling boundaries put around relationships? Might marriage be of less importance than our culture, from Christian fundamentalists to the Human Rights Campaign (HRC), wishes us to believe?

Clearly, the permissibility of and possibilities for polysexual polyamory form one category of questions raised by the existence of bisexuality. When we imagine the fluid, dynamic family and kinship units that could be created through such relationships, we begin to see the necessity of something much different than simply state-sanctioned monogamous unions. Ought the state to even be the arbiter of family? How might we meet the needs of every kind of partnership and family in our society, and might we do so outside the confines of the state?

When we inhabit an identity far outside of normative assumptions, we can begin to question assimilationist, mainstream gay narratives. Yes, a cis gay man or a cis lesbian woman can get married in some countries, adopt children, and live a life with access to many of the privileges afforded to straight monogamous couples. But does that advantage have much relevance to a young person grappling with a non-binary sexuality? Of what use is marriage to a homeless queer teen, a trans person who cannot access the hormonal treatments they need to live, or a newly out bisexual whose support networks have just crumbled? Even after we have achieved change such that no queer person lacks the resources and support they need, what meaning does the promise of a "normal" life have to a person who, whether in crisis or not, will always be so much more than just an assimilated, standardized, or "passing" identity?

If being gay is different from being straight (and I contend that it is, or should be), where does that leave non-monosexuals? Are we, too, different from straight people? Are we less different, more different, or just *differently* different than gay and lesbian people? Are we somewhat like gay people and somewhat like straight people?

If queerness is fundamentally different from straightness, non-monosexuals are just as different from heterosexuals as monosexual queer people—perhaps more so. The fact that our desire transcends gender or encompasses more than one gender suggests that we are not simply gayness-lite, or straightness plus something strange and uncertain. Bisexuality and other non-monosexual identities are marginalized, stigmatized, and erased precisely because they challenge assumptions surrounding sexuality, gender, and relationships. They smash stereotypes as they refuse to be shut up in binary boxes.

Introduction

What is a bisexual, polysexual, or pansexual like? There is no one right answer, and that is okay. There is no one right way to be or not be sexual, and there is no one right way to have or not have gender. We live in the gloriously rainbow space outside of categories. We should be the powerhouses and poster children of the queer movement, yet we are most often ignored in both mainstream cishet and gay narratives. If we aren't ignored, we are usually mocked or treated as posers who are "playing at gay" before we settle down to a happy, heterosexual life.

That is why this book is important: By compiling these diverse personal stories, we refuse to be dismissed. We require that society takes us as we are, without pigeonholes or labels except those we choose on our own authority. With unapologetic celebration of self-identification, this collection of writing challenges dominant, pervasive cultural narratives from beginning to end.

And so, the overthrow of controlled, stifling narratives about sexuality and gender starts here. In our own liberation lies the potential for the liberation of many others. When we are silenced, the world is presented with simple, discrete categories enforced by the elite. When we begin to speak, categories are broken down, and we are able to hear the rumblings of a greater revolution to come.

PART TWO: NARRATIVES

THE INVISIBLE B
By Faith Beauchemin

Being bisexual is freedom, and it is invisibility. I flip-flop between calling myself bisexual and pansexual. Bi is the word everyone knows, while pansexual doesn't leave anyone out. You see, I don't care what your gender is, or lack thereof. I'm attracted to people, not genders or genitals.

That doesn't mean I'm attracted to every single person, and it doesn't mean I have crushes on everyone I hang out with. It doesn't mean I'll go home with just anyone. All it means is that I could potentially be with a person who lies anywhere on or off the gender spectrum.

To be quite honest, I didn't know pansexuality even existed up until very recently. While I was growing up as a fundamentalist Christian, the "being gay is a choice" narrative sort of made sense to me. I mean, everyone had the ability to be attracted to everyone, right? I read a Christian modesty book that claimed everyone is "drawn to the female form" because it is just objectively beautiful. I figured I must be straight because I knew I was attracted to men, and since any pleasure I found in female beauty was purely "artistic," it had nothing at all to do with my sexuality. Besides, all the Christian dating books had a tiny appendix tucked in the back that warned of the dangers of "predatory college lesbians." So, I knew lesbianism existed, but all of my associations were totally negative.

The Invisible B

Even when I became less naïve, when I started thinking that people were born homosexual and understood that most gays and lesbians (like most straight people) are not predators, I still didn't realize that bisexuality existed. "Bicurious" was a term I was loosely aware of, but I thought it was a descriptor of an in-between phase, a transition between heterosexuality and homosexuality. Since I was definitely attracted to men, I knew I couldn't possibly be a lesbian. Simple as that. There was no other option. Monosexism was all I knew.

And that is what I mean when I say bisexuality is invisibility: As bisexuals, we get erased a lot. The biggest problem is what I term "Schrödinger's bisexual," which is when a person is perceived as either straight or gay depending on who they're in a relationship with. I'm dating a man right now, therefore everybody assumes I'm straight. Typically, bisexuality can't be determined by just one interaction with a person or by one specific point in time. It doesn't help matters that many people talk about bisexuals as though we are "switching" between heterosexuality and homosexuality.

Of course, as a woman I am sometimes permitted the total opposite of erasure—and that is performance. Men like the idea of a bisexual woman because their first thought is often of having a threeway. One night in a bar, a girl leaned over and kissed me. Immediately a man walked from across the room and asked, "Mind if I join in?" While visions of a porn-worthy fuckfest danced in his head, no doubt. Later, I tried to talk to a friend about how frustrating it is that no one thinks you're bi unless you've actually had a homosexual experience. He just jokingly spun a scenario where I and another woman would have sex and he would film it.

This reaction is part of the overarching issue of female sexuality being owned by men; if we are not having sex *with* them, we must at least be performing for their gaze. That's why most threesome porn is female-female-male, and why many men think that bisexual women exist only to have threesomes with them, or that lesbian women can be "cured" by their magical dicks. And that is all such bullshit. My sexuality—whatever it is—is mine and mine alone.

However, the seemingly fluid pansexual approach is all too often deemed everybody's property. More so than anyone else's, my sort of sexuality is approached with doubt. Everyone makes assumptions and speculates about the causes and motivations behind my sexuality (no, I am not just "greedy" and I am not going to try to fuck you. No, I am not disease-ridden or commitment-phobic. No, I'm not going to cheat on my partner).

Each time I field a question or assumption like this, it's a reminder of how truly queer-phobic our society remains. It is a society that will accept gay people—grudgingly, gradually—as long as they want to be just like straight people. Occasionally, trans people may find acceptance, but this is usually on the condition that they have had whatever surgery is deemed "necessary" for them to pass as cisgender. But anyone who is genderqueer, agender, or pansexual is met with flat-out denial of their self-identification: "You're lying," or "You just want attention."

Do I really though? No more than anyone else. I hate the fact that being honest about myself means I'll get extra attention. But we haven't reached a truly all-points-on-the-spectrum-accepting utopia yet. In fact, we're pretty far from it.

Actually admitting to myself that I was pansexual was truly liberating, though. It was just as liberating to learn that pansexuality exists. I used to fight my attraction to women, not so much because I thought it was "sinful"—although yes, the story of my sexuality is also concurrent to my deconversion—but because I thought if I gave in to that attraction, I would have to get rid of my attraction to men. It came as a great relief when I understood that it is possible, acceptable, and even normal to be attracted to all types of people. For the first time, I was no longer trying to fit my sexuality into a mold built by patriarchal society. I could like whatever and whomever I liked without feeling guilty or needing to repress anything.

So what's it like being pansexual? I'm not exactly sure. I've never been anything else. What's sexuality like for all of you out there who are monosexual?

Due to my circumstances and the timing of finally coming out to myself, I have never had sex with anyone but men. I've been in love with a few women, but didn't realize it at the time. It's not really a point of bitterness for me, though. I don't have to experience sex with all types of people to know my orientation (many people often know their sexual orientations before having sex of any kind). Right now, I'm happily in a relationship and I don't see that changing any time soon. If I die never having had sex with anyone but men, I won't feel like I was robbed, and I will still be pansexual.

Of course there is still much work to be done to make this world a better, more accepting place for those who are not heterosexual or cisgender. But coming out can be the first step. Coming out to yourself, to embrace your own freedom, and coming out to everyone else, to combat invisibility.

This is me taking that first step.

NOT STRAIGHT ...
OR ANYTHING ELSE FOR THAT MATTER
by Hugh Goldring

THERE IS ALREADY ONE GAY MARRIAGE IN MY IMMEDIATE FAMILY. I have every expectation that there will be another in the next few years, so let's break out the fancy cocktails and Erasure B-sides, already. In a lot of ways, gay marriage was the political issue I cut my teeth on as a baby activist, turning up at rallies to shout down the infamous Pastor Phelps, though he never had the decency to turn up anyway. But then, decency wasn't really his strong suit.

From the outside, my sexuality looks like a much more straightforward thing. I have had a long string of flings and committed relationships with women, settling finally into what is beginning to look suspiciously like a lifetime partnership with my darling Nicole. This is the story that I have generally preferred to put on display for public consumption; it's less work and maybe not for the reasons you might think.

It's not particularly a secret that I'm sexually attracted to men, insofar as I really understand "man" and "woman" to be static categories. In fact, I

Not Straight ... Or Anything Else For That Matter

am mostly taken in by tertiary sexual characteristics common to humans regardless of physiology: charm, tenderness, compassion and respect. When pressed for a description I'll usually tell people that I'm "omnivorous" or retreat into teenage cliché by protesting that labels are for tin cans. Again, that's easier than explaining, but explaining is exactly what I'll do here.

I doubt I'm letting any felines out of captivity when I say that *most men wouldn't know consent if it pepper sprayed them outside a nightclub.* Sadly, my experience is that this statement is true of men no matter who they want to fuck. It's my experience that I'm speaking for so please don't climb down my throat about "not all gay men," because not all the men in these stories are gay and it's not my problem anyway.

Let's begin at the beginning. When I was seventeen I had my first serious girlfriend. I wore skirts to high school because fuck you, that's why. Along with what I described as my bisexuality, my girlfriend was convinced that she could never trust me. I was always going to be "missing something" that she couldn't give to me, like if I didn't have a smorgasbord of genitalia to graze on, I would melt into a glassy puddle. I guess the following story didn't help.

She had a gay confidant. He took an interest in my Livejournal (a monument to my inanity that you'll never find, so don't go looking). He wanted to meet me and sent flattering messages to that effect. I was young, vain, and stupid. We met for dessert in the Byward Market in Ontario, where we exchanged adolescent musings on love, loss, and the meaning of life. He bought me pie. It was cold out but we went for a walk down into Strathcona Park. He had hand-knit a scarf. It kept my ears warm. He liked me. Like, *liked me* liked me. I had a girlfriend. He was her confidant, but she wasn't his, I guess, because "She doesn't need to know," he insisted, as his hand crept up my thigh. As his face drew close to mine. As every "no" that passed my lips only seemed to spur him on. These days, he works for a national student organization. I'll let you guess which one, but here's a clue: it's the one that loves lawsuits.

He was the first boy I ever kissed. Not because I really wanted to. It felt disloyal. But because he made me feel sorry for him, and guilty, like I owed him something that I was withholding out of a perverse sense of spite. I didn't feel like, "Hey, I have a partner and I told you no repeatedly—get the fuck out of my face." I didn't have a framework to do that in. I knew what it was like to long to be touched. So I didn't want to touch him, but at least I could do something for him. He had made that abundantly clear.

My older brother was newly out of the closet. When he heard this story, he chose to respond by telling me that I didn't have to kiss men just because he did. It's hard for me to describe in words how shitty and invalidating it felt to hear what I know was only a thoughtless quip. Along with the experience surrounding the kiss, that response threaded together two of the longest strands in my attraction to men. When they desired me, men would pursue physical contact insistently, even aggressively. When I expressed my ambiguous feelings around this interplay of desire and disrespect, my sexuality would be dismissed, defined, policed. It was a piece of my sexuality that I was going to have to fight for. I'm sorry to say at that point I had chosen surrender.

I lived in residence with two openly gay men. One of them was a friend, but I was leery of getting too close. I didn't totally understand why I balked at his invitation to sneak a bottle of wine into a movie theater at a time when I was all about that kind of shit. Seems pretty obvious in hindsight—I had already learned to be afraid of men's interest in me. He was actually a sweetheart. Or maybe he just figured I was straight; certainly the other gay guy who lived in residence had come to that conclusion.

"He says he's bisexual but he hasn't slept with either of us," this fine specimen of a human being remarked to my friend (the other openly gay guy in residence). He couldn't get his head around the idea that I might be too picky to fuck two whole dudes. I doubt he could have figured out that I might be afraid of being touched, grabbed, kissed against my will. Afraid that once again my "no" would be interpreted as "try harder." That was all too complicated, I guess. I wouldn't fuck them, so I was a faker. Maybe it's not an easy thing to understand.

Later, when I was living with an ex, she came home from the bar with a gay male friend. I was sober but tortured and sought to dissolve myself in physical contact with both of them. When I felt in control it was a comfort, or at least an anesthetic. At a certain point I think my ex felt that a line had been crossed and she withdrew. Before I knew how to react, her friend reassured her, "That's okay. You don't have to do anything you don't want to. Hugh will fuck me in the ass. You can watch."

My turn to stiffen, to recoil. He could register her discomfort and respect her boundaries because she wasn't an object of interest. But the idea that this proposed sex act would require my input, much less my consent, didn't seem to occur to him. I fled, sliding into safety behind huge oak double doors. Shut in my room, I tried to make sense of what had happened. I hadn't put the pieces together when he started yanking on the door rollers, trying to force them open. I froze, helpless in bed, as he forced his way into my room. He was drunk, enormous, apologetic. My ex was with him. He was sorry and good hearted, but didn't understand why making assumptions about my consent was scary to me—never mind the sound of him forcing his way into my room for a conversation I wasn't ready to have. He also thought he could talk me into coming back out and picking up where we'd left off. Forgive my cynicism but, "Are you okay?" doesn't sound as sincere when the clear subtext is "Chill out so I can fuck you."

That experience put the whole same-sex thing on ice for a while. My next girlfriend was convinced that even my straightest friends were secretly angling to fuck me. While that was flattering, I'm afraid that my raw animal magnetism is more of a cooked animal carcass; in other words, they weren't biting. Again, I didn't help matters by speculating that her best friend must be gay, and by kissing an army captain in front of her. I guess when he caressed my thighs under the table of the pub while maintaining eye contact with her, to assert dominance, it may have given her cause for concern.

The next thing that stands out in my little chronicle of consent is an interaction at an activist event. I'd been on my feet eighteen hours a day for weeks, and my back was way beyond the "sore" that I complain about when I am desperate for some pretext for human contact. It ached something awful. I went into a tent with a more experienced activist, who was urbane, cute, funny. He was a hothouse flower in the social justice spotlight. I felt lucky to attract his attention. He always seemed to be in front of a crowd or camera, his name on the lips of everyone I looked up to in the community. He had been leaning on me all night at an emergency meeting.

He didn't ask before he straddled me, but sometimes that's just the mark of an extremely capable masseur. I was sore, tired and beyond vulnerable. I was prepared to let it pass. But when he started grinding his pelvis into my ass—well, that was less ambiguous. I was confident enough to protest, to indicate I wasn't interested in anything sexual. It could have felt like a breakthrough. It didn't.

"I don't know what you're talking about."

Maybe our bodies were speaking different languages, but if I grind my pelvis into someone, it means that I am either initiating sexual contact or goofing around with some very old, very straight friend. He acted like it was no big deal. The backrub stopped. He didn't feel compelled to explain himself, much less apologize. I was frustrated, confused, disempowered. I hadn't been pressured into anything, sure, but I felt like I was the crazy one. Whatever the reality of the situation, by refusing to acknowledge that he'd crossed my boundaries without seeking consent, he took a large part of my power away. It felt like I'd just been told "No one will believe you, so don't bother saying anything."

Of course, I've got a mouth that could swallow the moon. So I told plenty of people. I guess that was around the time I began to have a supportive community of people—inevitably women—who could help me contextualize these experiences. They didn't tell me I was "asking for it." They didn't call me a tease or roll their eyes at what others might have assumed was one more phony bi attention whore who got what was coming to him. That meant a hell of a lot. Still does.

The following year, I was riding in a cramped car that reeked of cigarettes and the irrepressible charm of an international documentarian of mystery. Also present was a locally infamous gay activist best known for self-anointing as an ally. I guess that was only one item on a long list of ordinations he felt qualified to perform, because the one cock I'd sucked wasn't enough for him to believe that I identified as "queer." The term had a comfortable fluidity to it. By that point I had been with people whose sexuality was less of a ticked box, and more of an expository paragraph with light pencil sketches. I had begun to understand some of the ways in which my own sexual identity was complicated by the politics of consent, of gender performance and mental illness. "Bisexual" hadn't fit for a long time, and just when I thought I could fit the tufts of my disheveled hair into the many-jeweled prongs of the "queer" tiara, this arrogant prick snatched it off my brow and ground it under one metaphorically high-heeled foot. It was queeny in the worst sense of the word, and sweetie, you know how anarchists feel about monarchy.

It wasn't the last experience like that. Recently, another gay comrade at a party told me I didn't fit the bill and I just said "fair enough." I can take a hint. I can pass as straight so I don't get to be proud. That's okay. As Groucho

Not Straight ... Or Anything Else For That Matter

Marx says, I would never join a club that cares where I stick my member. So I gave up on queer and got evasive when people asked about my sexuality. If you're clever enough, people don't realize that your stonewall wit is really a thin gauze over all-but-open wounds. No one wants to hear about all the times you—a man—have had your boundaries violated; that's what I had figured, anyway. Certainly no one thought it was a good excuse for why I didn't put out.

If there was a nail in the coffin of not wanting to get nailed, that nailing happened a few summers ago. I went out dancing with a friend and his perennial crush, who brought along her charming gay roomie. He was a small-town splash of cottage country lake water in a muscle shirt. But he had the coy cosmopolitanism of a country boy made good, and since he also had a boyfriend I figured it was safe to dance. Safe for everyone else, at least—you don't want to see my dance flails (I hesitate to call them moves).

When he suggested we all go back to their house for pomegranate mojitos, how could I resist? Their place was on my way and I never say no to a well-mixed cocktail. Soon we were like mint and pomegranate in his backyard hammock, cuddling and watching the sun come up around 5 AM. I snuggled into his shoulder and told him that he made me feel safe. I told him how often men had ignored my boundaries and treated me like a prize. I said in all the words I had—that's a lot of words, for those of you following along at home—that I was so *grateful* that he wasn't trying to fuck me. "Hey, thanks for not being a rapist."

It seems pathetic in hindsight, but that's where I was at, in not so many words. I was pitifully grateful to be held and treated tenderly by a man whom I found attractive. I felt like I might finally be evaluated for my personality first and my sexual availability only later. Plus, he had a boyfriend. What could possibly go wrong when he asked if I wanted to sleep over? Besides, he couldn't have been clearer: "We can just sleep."

God, finally. I could feel my heart melting just enough to admit that maybe I was ready to consider being involved in a sexual relationship with a man, if only I could find a queer single guy as decent as this dude. With an intoxicating mixture of trust, longing and opening up, it was the kind of hallelujah breakthrough that the movies rarely nail.

That is, until we climbed into bed and he rubbed his hard-on against my thigh for the better part of ten minutes before finally giving up. Surprise! Even after explicitly telling me that I could sleep over and he wouldn't try anything, the first thing that this upstanding model of respect and consent did was strip off his jeans and rub his stiff cock against my exposed flesh. But this time I knew better than to say anything; I didn't want to hear whatever shit he was going to feed me. I just waited for it to be over. I honestly think that if he'd kept at it long enough I would have slept with him just to get it over with.

The most horrible part was that it turned me on. Even as I felt disgusted, disappointed, verging on heartbroken, my body reacted. My consent was a border crossed so regularly that my nausea couldn't completely quell arousal. I breathed an inward sigh of relief when he stopped, and crept out into the dawn as soon as he was asleep. Later that same week I went out for drinks with my supportive lady pals. I told them this story. They all had a similar one—no, several similar ones. Christ, men are pigs.

So here's the point, if it ain't at all apparent. I love people, and for that reason, I love fucking. When it creates a moment of intimacy, a temporary teardown of barriers, that's bliss. I want to be able to feel that way with anyone I have chemistry with. I want to be able to feel that with men. But I don't generally fuck queer men because in my experience, "no" just means "try harder," and "stop that" is an invitation to gaslight me. Explaining at length that respecting my boundaries earns my trust apparently writes "fuck me" across my thigh in legible glitter. So yeah, I don't generally fuck men because I don't trust them not to try to rape me. I don't trust them to think that maybe *that's* the reason that I don't fuck men, even though I'm attracted to them. I guess it's easier to climb into the tree fort and shout, "no fake queers allowed" than it is to accept what a problem sexual aggression is *whenever* men are involved.

These aren't all my stories about sexually aggressive men. Just the ones that I have curated into a cozy museum of disrespected autonomy. These also aren't all my stories about gay men policing the boundaries of my sexual identity. I haven't bothered to talk about the shitty way people like me are often discussed in queer media and pop culture at large.

I also haven't talked about my own history as a sexually aggressive man. So, full disclosure—in past relationships with women, I have done things every bit as bad as the men in these stories, and worse. That's the subject of another article. I'm holding off on writing it because I am still not sure what to say about it. For now, let me just say that toxic masculinity is an intoxicant as well as a poison. It teaches you to understand human relationships in terms of power, and to see them as successful when you get what you want without giving up more than you'd like. This is a lethal attitude, I know. I am going to spend the rest of my life flushing it out of my system.

But let's not end on that note. It's not the whole story. Not all my experiences are bad. Here's a good one: When I was in university I had a dear male friend. We made out at parties. We flirted and bickered like reluctant fiancés. I fantasized about him and pretended he drove me crazy, when really I would have liked to get him alone. Other than smoking a barrel of cigarettes between lectures and having some hella questionable politics, he essentially defined what I thought of as an attractive man.

Near the end of university, we were joking around about "experimenting in college." We teased out the prospect of sleeping together. What would we do? Who would we tell and how would we tell them? We were delighted by the scandal of the whole thing. At least on my end, that was a convenient veil to throw over the deeper feelings that lingered with the longing to be physical.

So, when we made sure we both wanted it, when we had an understanding, we went to it. He was a lot more experienced than I was. He was gentle, guiding but never forceful. He was cautious, thoughtful, clear in his needs and boundaries. I felt comfortable to do the same. I won't elaborate, but suffice to say I still blush when I think about it. Afterwards we took a shower together and nuzzled there in the shower. Then we laid down in bed and cuddled. We haven't done it again, but I think half of that has been a question of timing. He has given me every reason to trust him, and *that* is the space where I am open to intimacy with men. I'm not sorry about it because it is fucking beautiful, like skipping stones on a still lake on the last day of your life. I'll take that over pomegranate mojitos any day.

So, no—I'm not bi. There is no binary. I'm apparently not queer either, as I haven't sucked enough dicks to get my card punched as a Political Queer™. With a lifetime of crushes, deep romantic feelings, kisses and sexual fantasies about men, I'm sure as hell not straight. I guess you could say I'm a lover. I love people, no matter what they have going on between their legs, if they give me the space to do so. Sounds a lot less shitty than "omnivorous," doesn't it? Maybe I'll stick with it.

FLYING IN THE FACE OF EVERYTHING
By Kierstyn King

I'VE ALWAYS TRIED TO FLY UNDER THE RADAR, to exist in the shadows, and to be invisible. I spent my entire childhood perfecting that skill, trying to go as unnoticed by my parents as I could, because being noticed always ended up going over poorly for me.

Simultaneously, it's all I've ever wanted and needed—to be noticed. Sometimes I'm bothered by the fact that I am so good at becoming invisible, even though there is a safety in it.

I'm a married, bisexual, non-binary agnostic with no kids and no desire to have them.

Every bit of that last sentence (well, except the married part) flies in the face of everything I was raised to be.

Growing up, I didn't know that bisexuality (or anything besides gay and straight) was a thing; the concept of being transgender was scoffed at and passed off as fake. I was assigned female at birth and raised to be a good Christian home-schooled girl, I missed out on opportunities I would have otherwise been interested in, or have later found out that I'm good at, because of being born with female genitalia.

I was told that my glory was to be feminine, and get married to a suitably masculine man, and have oodles of children, and be a good little housewife who never did anything more interesting than crochet, cook, and homeschool. Despite the amount of everything telling me that was what I should be and do and like, I never did. I never felt particularly "feminine" or like a girl—but I never felt particularly like a boy, either, though my more "masculine" tendencies did lead to years of feeling broken because I wasn't "supposed to" feel that way.

My parents tried to tell me that "being a girl is just better" because life is supposedly so much easier for women (who don't have any independence).

I was supposed to be content being a helpless damsel—not become a protector.

It wasn't until recently that I stopped feeling broken because of who I am. It wasn't until recently that I had words to describe how I felt, or more accurately, didn't feel. I don't really know how to explain what it feels like to grow up feeling wrong or broken for something that's innately *you*, something that you can't fix but are told is wrong and not normal or acceptable.

It took me a long time to admit to myself that I was bi. In actuality I'm pansexual—gender isn't really a thing I notice or take into account. I call myself bi because that takes less explaining, and I tend to opt for what's most easily understood.

I had a lot of awkward moments as a teenager when I would notice people's faces and like them, only to realize that they belonged to girls and I quickly buried those moments with shame, fear, and guilt.

The thing about being sheltered and also heaped with guilt and anxiety around being impure or lustful is that even though I masturbated and felt that was wrong, I reasoned I wasn't really lusting because I was fantasizing primarily about girls (I only knew of gays, lesbians didn't exist). I had a guy in there as wallpaper, but he was just sort of … fully dressed and I wasn't really into my imaginary dude as much … or at all.

I spent a lot more time thinking about female bodies than male bodies. I never thought that was weird, but I never, ever said anything about it either. It wasn't until I came to understand myself as a bi/pansexual that all of those parts of my childhood and adolescence suddenly made sense. It wasn't until I was able to give names to how I felt or didn't feel that I started being able to express and accept myself. Before that I just felt this vague sense of being different and wrong, faking my way through normalcy even though it killed me inside.

I came out as bisexual publicly on my blog in 2013. I didn't hear anything directly from my family, but I heard through the grapevine that they flipped out and decided, yet again, that I was doomed to hell. My sisters unfriended me—at the demand of my parents, no doubt—shortly after my family got word. On vacation with my in-laws that summer, I learned that my bisexuality was a cause of great distress to my mother-in-law, who said, "Not that she was questioning my faithfulness or anything," and apparently spent nights crying over it.

I've felt judged by the people I'm related to by blood and by law for my existence—I'm not the delicate, submissive woman they wanted me to be, I'm not straight, and I don't know what the fallout will be if or when they learn that not only am I not feminine enough, but also I don't identify as a woman.

Rejecting the idea of traditional "gender roles" happened hand in hand with embracing my sexuality and realizing that my spouse and I are humans, not robots. This eventually lead to acceptance of all the ways I didn't fit in the boxes to which I'd been assigned (and hated). I was finally able to slowly start unpacking the tangled mess that is my gender identity. "The Genderbread Person," and Sam Killerman's TEDx talk, "The Complexities of Gender," were some of the first things I discovered that really helped shed some light on what is still a fluid, sometimes confusing process of figuring out who I am and what that means.

When I tell people about my sexuality or my gender identity, or that I have lady-sex with a friend sometimes, I either find a lot of support and understanding and it's beautiful—or I run into people who think I'm into anyone and should totally tell them everything about what it's like to have had sex with both a male and a female at different times. There are also the people who find passive-aggressive ways to imply that I'm lesser, broken, or just bitter because I'm neither womanly nor do I consider myself a woman.

My existence seems to break the brains of people who don't understand the concept of life outside the binary or in the middle of the rainbow; people who still think women should like "womanly things," or want children, and maybe if they don't they're just not with the right partner, or bitter, or rejecting their nature—as opposed to embracing it.

Sometimes people don't seem to understand that standing outside the "norm"—outside the role society and my home environment arbitrarily decided I was to fulfill because of my genitalia—is not done because of some weird spite or spiritual issue or rebellion. It's done because this is my authentic self. It's a hard, vulnerable place to be in when people look at me and see everything they think I should be but am not, instead of seeing *just me*, a fellow human.

See, the thing is, occasionally I do like to paint my nails, and sometimes I want to make a loaf of bread and then eat it all myself because bread is my favorite food group—but these occaisonal expressions of traditional femininity don't define me or who I am as a human being who lives and loves, who has human traits and doesn't want to have to classify them as manly or womanly. Because they're just *human*, and humans are all different.

It hurts to feel unaccepted or misunderstood by family, friends, and society at large. Sometimes it gets overwhelming. But learning to accept myself and embrace whatever it means to be me—to be human, and fluid, and alive—is so much more freeing than trying to shut down all the parts of me that never fit in the boxes I was given.

Being myself—and finding out what that means—is hard, but it's worth it. It's a battle I'm willing to fight.

(UN)SEEN
By J.

I'M PANSEXUAL, AND I'M FRUSTRATED. Let me explain.
"I don't mean this to be disrespectful, but is that a thing? I mean, does the medical and psychological professional community recognize that as real?" That's what my brother asked me when I told him I was pansexual. It's not surprising, really, because in my experience most people don't know what pansexuality is, and as a conservative christian[1] evangelical, my brother certainly didn't either. (Yeah, ask me how the rest of *that* conversation went.)

"Wow, that's so cutting-edge. But I'm not surprised; you always were advanced." I heard that from a friend when I outed myself to her. I didn't know how to respond. Cutting-edge? Advanced? These words imply that others' orientations are old-fashioned, and I'm pretty sure sexuality doesn't become obsolete.

---

1   I intentionally don't capitalize christian because while I recognize that more progressive forms of christianity are more welcoming of the LBGTQ community, the bigoted sect I came from does not and to me does not deserve the respect of capitalization. — J.

"That's so utopian," an acquaintance remarked after she Googled pansexuality. Really? I don't think pansexuality is the ideal sexual orientation—*because there's not one*. However an individual identifies is just fine. I definitely don't want anyone to think I'm inferior, but I'm assuredly not superior either.

Likewise, there's the standard heteronormative remarks we all probably hear. After a recent snowstorm, a colleague sympathized with my complaints about spending an hour shoveling out my car: "Yeah, you don't have a husband to do it for you." First of all, I'm quite capable of clearing snow by myself; I just don't have to enjoy it. Second, I'm open to partnering with anyone regardless of gender, sex, or sexual orientation, so it is quite presumptive to mourn my lack of a husband. I'm confident that a chick or a trans* person can handle a shovel just as well as a cisgender, straight male!

These types of responses and off-hand remarks remind me that I have no place in heterosexual culture. They demonstrate how little the general public (including those of a progressive persuasion) understands pansexuality. Many have never even heard the term, and so I am constantly explaining myself. Another friend observed that folks with uncommon medical conditions often find themselves explaining their diseases. But pansexuality—like all orientations on the spectrum—isn't an illness. I'm not searching for a cure. I'm looking for a place to belong.

I don't fit in the straight world, but is there a place at the table for me in the LGBTQ community? After all, there is no "P" in the initialism. A lot of the time that's okay, because I'll embrace the Q. Yet, when I see the term LGBT, I wonder where someone like me belongs. When events are advertised as a "lesbian group" or a "bisexual gathering," I question if I would be welcomed. I suspect others who identify from a space within the middle of the spectrum do too.

Even as I type this, I fear people's responses. Who am I to critique the LGBT community, when it has only been within the past few years that I've stepped out of the straight shadows and identified myself as a member? But it has also been within the past few years that I have found my voice, so it is important for me to use it.

Let me explain. I've recently liberated myself from christian fundamentalism. For most of my life, I sincerely believed the dogma that forced me to disown myself in order to embrace God. Not only did I have to repress my sexuality as a woman and especially as a queer woman, but I had to silence all other aspects of who I was. This lasted up until a few years ago, when painful events and a PhD program opened my eyes to reality. I realized I could not reconcile the misogyny of evangelicalism with feminism. I could not blend fundamentalist absolutism with the T(t)ruth of postmodernism. So I walked away from religion. Some might say I lost my faith, but I believe I found myself. And with that came the legitimacy of my sexuality.

Accepting my pansexuality wasn't difficult. What I find challenging is wondering whether or not others will accept me. As a cisgender woman, I've experienced marginalization. What other types of oppression might I encounter as I embrace the social identity of an *atheist, pansexual woman*?

To heterosexual society, I appear as a lipstick-wearing, high-heel-walking, solely-male-loving woman. I probably look the same to the LGBTQ community. How does my "P" fit in? Where is the nuance I represent? In both spheres, I'm invisible.

WHAT YOU SEE ISN'T WHAT YOU GET
By Lucas

"I THOUGHT YOU WERE TOTALLY STRAIGHT," Connor said between kissing me and running his warm hands over my body. "This is like a dream fucking come true." I wish my too-actively politicalized brain hadn't ruined it for me when I thought to myself as I pressed against him, "This is being bi. They don't see you as you are until you do something about it." My brain *would* latch onto ideas of bisexual erasure instead of focusing on the awesome time I was supposed to be having in that moment.

In the thirteen years since I first told at least myself that I was bi, I have had only serious relationships with women, and the vast majority of my sexual encounters have been with women as well. It often gets me questioning my own label of bisexual and how honest that label may be. I could just be a straight dude (and judging by all my relationship partners, I am) who can understand the idea of sexual attraction to another dude. From the outside, it looks like I could easily erase the idea that I am attracted to men, or have been in the past. That's the so-called "bisexual privilege": That we can pass for straight, if only we wanted to. And why wouldn't you choose to be straight if you could? Wouldn't that be grand?

Of course, the idea of *choosing* one's sexuality is anathema in queer and progressive communities. But somehow it's more acceptable when applied to those who identify as bisexual or pansexual instead of those who identify as gay or lesbian, as long as the so-called "choice" points in a direction that "makes it easier for you to not look queer." That odd double standard for bi folk creates a mistrust about us, emanating from both straight people and gay people. That much communal mistrust, it feeds into a fundamental mistrust of myself: am I *really* bisexual?

On our first and only date, after a long draw on his cigarette, Connor asked me, "So, what's your deal? Everyone thinks you're straight." And with that, I had been given this opportunity to talk out my sexuality to a real, receptive, respectful person. I tried to explain to him how I identify as bisexual, but my attractions haven't been the 50/50 split that the word implies; how it surprises me to this day when I find myself attracted to more than just women. It was a lot to throw out on a first date, but hey, he asked. Maybe he thought the stressed-out rambling I was doing looked cute.

I can't help but wonder how Connor took all that, since only hours later I called off any potential future dating. Sometimes I wonder now if I'm still afraid of the part of me that also finds men attractive, and though smoking is an additional dealbreaker for me, if that fear wasn't also a part of why I closed myself off from him. Or rather, why I closed myself off from myself. Again.

There's a common retort among secret bigots: "Hey man, look, I don't care if you're a gay or whatever, just *don't shove it in my face.*" As just about every person could, at first blush, pass as straight (and the default assumption is always *straight*), that argument really comes down to, "Make sure you *never identify yourself as you wish to be*, for my personal comfort is more important." Pride parades, as flamboyant as they can be (and flamboyant they have every right to be), are necessary because of that kind of half-baked, bigoted reasoning. Queer representation in the media is necessary. Identifying myself as bi is necessary, because it's who I am. Visibility is important, because that's how I feel anyone exists in this society. Erasure is as good as death.

But what does visibility look like for me? Can I just go out with a guy and hold his hand and fall in love with him without it being a politicized event? Is there such a thing as visibility of non-standard, transgressive sexuality that doesn't involve a trade-off of safety and security? I can't blame Connor for his thinking I was straight. Maybe I can blame society for building these assumptions, but what is that worth? And how can I address the visibility of my sexuality when I still get confused and surprised by it? What can I do about the *political* if the *personal* is still so hard to confront?

Only recently have I been more casually open about my sexuality, when I think I am safe to do so. I've told a few co-workers, somewhat nonchalantly, when the topic has come up. Working in theatre as I do, jobsite conversations tend to be lax and informal. But even still, there are times when people who I thought would be more sensitive about queer sexualities say something that only serves to highlight how little they know about bisexuality. Once, in regards to my sexuality, my openly gay roommate said, "You're into *everything*!" Every space becomes a little less safe when "jokes" like that pass through. There are only so many times I can roll my eyes before I would rather roll myself up in a sleeping bag and hide forever.

And there are still very unsafe spaces, like that which my family inhabits. While visiting relatives over a summer holiday, one of my uncles asked me if I had a girlfriend back in Philadelphia. And I said, in a joking tone so I could rescue myself if I needed to, "No, no girlfriend. No boyfriend." His reaction, his so *very* expected reaction, was, "What, boyfriend? I *hope* you don't have a boyfriend!" I bailed out with a muttered, "Just joking." A few hours later, another uncle asked the insipid and harmful question, "When do straight people get to be 'proud?'" I was only drunk enough to say, "Straight people get to be proud all the damn time," but luckily not drunk enough to angrily come out to them. And so, as they haven't earned the right to know me, they never will. Maybe this will pay off in terrible dividends in the future, but when I'm around them, my trust in myself plummets, and they are in no way going to help me stop falling.

With this much mistrust coming from the outside, I'm fighting the internal battle to trust myself: that I really *am* bisexual, that this much is true about me. I should trust that it is true when I look at a hot guy on the bus and think "Oh, he's a really hot guy on the bus, and here I am looking at how hot he is." Some days are easier than others, and they get easier when I don't have to *confront* my sexuality but can just *be* with it. I have to trust myself when so many other people don't even trust the *idea* of myself. If I'm to do anything with any visibility at all, I have to see myself as I am.

I COULD PICK A SIDE ... BUT I WON'T
By Liam H. Smith

I AM BISEXUAL. I can and do become attracted to women, men, and people of other genders. I find it incredibly, ridiculously hard to actually say so.

Because I have a whole ton of internalized biphobia. Because, despite evidence to the contrary, I'm forever looking for clues that I'm somehow "really" hetero or "really" gay. Because I live in a world that bases sexual identity on the relation between someone's gender and the gender of their partners, and then tries to fit everyone into "straight" and "gay".

Gender preferences don't seem to be a fixed thing for me. I very, very consistently find people with darker hair more attractive than people with blonde hair. I very consistently find other autistic people more attractive than neurotypical people. I currently seem to find men generally more attractive than women, but this has changed rapidly and I fully expect it to change again.

Yet I never quite feel "bi enough" to call myself bisexual. Even when I was dating a man, a nonbinary person *and* a woman, I didn't feel "bi enough" because I was mainly attracted to women. Now, I'm attracted to a lot of men and in a long term relationship with a woman I am very much in love with and very, very attracted to. And I don't feel "bi enough".

I Could Pick a Side ... But I Won't

I think this has a lot to do with the constant pressure, both overt and covert, to "pick a side." The world around me and a heck of a lot of the people that comprise it make it very clear that I may like either women or men. Pick one. I may be straight, and if I can't be straight then I should be gay. Pick a side. Circle one option only.

And as a bisexual, I could choose to be straight. Both the straight community and the LG community push the message that no one would ever choose to be gay if they had the choice. Yet both tell me that I do have the choice. Pick a side. The conclusion is obvious: I'm supposed to choose to be "straight."

Leaving aside the difficulty that cis people have with understanding how "gay" and "straight" work for trans people such as myself (put simply, any relationship I have with a cis person will be seen as "gay" by a large number of people), what would it mean for me to pick a side and choose to be "straight"?

I know I can't force myself to stop feeling attracted to other men. I don't imagine I could force myself to not fall in love with them, either. I could, at least in theory, choose not to pursue relationships with men. I could stop flirting with men. Stop checking them out. Stop smiling at pretty guys. Maybe. It'd take a whole heap of effort on my part. It'd hurt.

And I know I can't see gender identity. I'd have to avert my attention from anyone I thought *might* be a man. I'd have to hypocritically dump any partner who discovered themselves to also be a trans man.

I'd become distant in my friendships with other men. I'd probably leave the LGBT community out of fear of "giving away" that I am bi. I'd become more anxious, expecting my mannerisms or too-long glances to give away that I like men. I'd feel constantly under surveillance, and detached and alienated from straight male friends.

Even more important than all that, though, I'd resent myself. I'd know that I was cutting myself off from wonderful people, and for what? So people around me can feel comfortable about boxing everyone into "gay" and "straight"?

I would miss out on relationships that could have been. Picking one side means rejecting the other side, after all. There may be men out there who could love me immensely. Men who could show me the world in ways I have never seen it before. Men who could inspire me to be the very best person

I could be. There may be men out there with whom I could share awesome sex. Men whom I might never want to stop kissing. Men who would hold me while I cry, and just as willingly help me choose what to make for dinner. Men whom I could love, trust, respect, and care for. There are women like that out there too, of course, but choosing to pretend to be straight would cut me off from the potential of those men and deny us a chance to love each other. I cannot help but see it as an act of great emotional violence to ask me to do this to myself and to those men.

It would be similarly harmful to ask me to choose to be "gay." To deny that I love, have loved, and can love women. To steel my heart and avert my eyes from people I could love, just because my perception of their gender says I *ought* not choose not to love them? It's an unthinkably terrible thing to do to yourself.

And that's what "picking a side" really means. It means denying yourself the possibility of relationships with people because you're afraid of "looking gay" or of "stealing straight privilege." It means being so afraid of people thinking you've "changed sides" that you let yourself lose out on potential happiness, just to look consistent. Just to hold up the very system of monosexism that is crushing you.

In my experience, bi people are much more likely than lesbian, gay or heterosexual people to have anxiety problems. Some people think the constant covert and overt pressure to "pick a side" is part of the reason for this. I already have anxiety problems. I don't want to add, "What if people think I'm gay?" to them, thanks very much.

I am bisexual. I'm still struggling, seven years after coming out to myself, to accept that fact and be okay with it. I am saying, here and now, that I will never, ever choose to "pick a side." There are too many wonderful people in the world whom I could love and who could love me. I will not deny myself a chance to love and be loved by someone simply because of their gender.

CALL THE DOCTOR
By M.

Acknowledging your bisexuality can be a little tricky in a country where seemingly nobody knows or cares what bisexuality means.

India. I live in India: not the most progressive country in the world. I'm privileged enough that my friends aren't terrible homophobes, I'm not taught that homosexuality is a sin, and it probably won't be a big deal if I come out. But with the recent ruling on Section 377 (which specifies that "unnatural" sexual acts are illegal), and with a right-wing government coming into power, it's not exactly a welcoming environment. There is no representation of queer or genderqueer people on television, and the premise of the only recent mainstream Bollywood movie to addressed homosexuality, *Dostana*, was that two boys pretended to be lovers in order to jump an airplane or something—I don't even know. They ridiculed the whole concept and used tired stereotypes instead of actually starting a meaningful dialogue. I do know that the onscreen kiss wasn't received very well. It has been years since then, but it's still not a pretty topic to bring up.

I was fifteen when I first noticed my attraction to girls. It confused and scared the hell out of me. I kept thinking that it was wrong, that I was supposed to like only boys, that something was wrong with me—*maybe I'll grow out of it, I hope I grow out of it, am I a freak, I don't want to be a freak, why me, it's just a phase, no it isn't just a phase, it doesn't matter whether or not it's a phase but I should probably keep this to myself.* There was no one and nothing telling me that it was wrong, but I guess in a world where being accepted is still a fight, that is the default setting.

I'm seventeen now. It took a year and a half to get to the stage where I don't mind being attracted to girls. Where I've come out to a couple of friends. Where if someone asks me about being attracted to girls, I won't deny it. Of course, that doesn't mean my entire life is centered around an attraction to girls. Nor does it mean I don't like guys.

I'm still confused about the difference between bisexual and pansexual. But at this point, when I'm still trying to figure out my identity and place in the world, and when labels are unnecessary and sometimes detrimental, it doesn't matter much. At this point what matters is that I am comfortable with who I am, and I can give advice to anyone who asks for it. It took a lot to get here.

It took a lot of books—especially a biography of Natalie Barney, one of the first "out" lesbians—all read on a Kindle so my parents wouldn't find out what I was reading. It took a lot of Citizen Radio, a political humour podcast that also says it's okay to be who you are, as long as you're not as asshole. It took a lot of spoken-word poetry, especially by Andrea Gibson and Denice Frohman, and a lot of riot grrrl music—especially Sleater-Kinney's *Call The Doctor*, which addressed my "Something's wrong with me, call the doctor!" feeling. It took a lot of tears, a lot of tea, and a lot of time. I may seem like a hysterical little girl to all the older people reading this, but at times it seemed like these things were my only friends.

The biggest realization to come out of this, is that we need a more accepting mainstream media that can foster a more accepting mindset in people. And I focus on "mainstream," because not everyone has access to books, podcasts, or '90s punk music. Not everyone is able to have their voice heard like this, and not everyone can be comfortable with their own voice, in their own skin.

With the Supreme Court now recognizing people of a third gender, but still upholding Section 377—written when the British ruled over us—there has been a bit of conversation on alternate orientations and identities, but it's far from perfect. The conversation isn't intersectional at all, which means that mentally, we're still in our gated communities and won't really get to discuss anything with someone who doesn't share our view. The conversation between educated upper-class people is not quite the same as that among poor or religious people. This is going to be a major problem.

Prime Minister Modi has served for a long time in the Rashtriya Swayamsevak Sangh, a right-wing Hindu nationalist group and the Bharatiya Janata Party (BJP)'s ideological parent, that has expressed a zero-tolerance policy for homosexuality, although there is hope they will soften their stance. Rajnath Singh, the Minister for Home Affairs, has said it is "unnatural." This political environment is definitely not as dire as some other countries, but it isn't very welcoming either.

All that we can do now is talk about it, write about it, scream about it. When we educate ourselves, preach acceptance where we can and tolerance where we can't. Being educated and tolerant is not the same as being accepting. If I go out right now and say I'm gay, bisexual, or pansexual most people will say that's alright, but half of them won't talk to me again. There is nowhere to turn, though a lot of advertisements today are socially conscious and trying to foster an environment for positive dialogue. It will still take a while. If there was a gay character on any major TV show today, there would be enormous controversy surrounding it. As much as it pains me to write this, I think social acceptance will have to come before legal acceptance, and both are a long way off. I'm sure there is queer-focused independent media here, but I haven't found any yet. I've had to look to the fringes of another culture to find representation. There's always hope, though, that writers, musicians, comedians, and actors—and most importantly, the amazing activists—will continue changing mindsets, moving towards a more accepting society.

Being comfortable and open about being bisexual (among social circles—it's still not something I would discuss with my family) means that all the energy that went into my doubt and anger and self-hate, can now be directed into more productive things, even if it's just fighting with someone who insists on using the term "faggot" derogatorily, or having a talk with a friend's younger sister who is in the same place I was in two years back. It's not that I am a worldly expert, or even someone who gives very good advice. But sometimes an open discussion can help one person, and that person can help two people, and those two people can help four people—it's a snail's pace, but at least it's movement.

Unfortunately, even with the ruling on the third gender, the dialogue in India is going to exclude bisexual, pansexual, transgender, agender, and genderqueer people for a few years. As much as I'd like to make the dialogue more inclusive, homosexuality is the most understood and easily digestible out of all of those terms, and has the most direct legal repercussions. We definitely don't have it as bad as countries like Russia or Nigeria, but there are so many issues we need to deal with first (poverty, education and the like) that a decent mainstream dialogue, let alone a marriage equality bill, is going to take a lot of time and effort.

But we'll reach a point one day when being non-cisgender and non-heterosexual will not have the social and legal implications it has today. It won't be a big deal to talk about attraction to someone of the same sex—love, relationships, all of that. It won't be a big deal to sidestep the gender binary; maybe we won't have a gender binary. Maybe there won't be a need for projects like this, because voices like ours won't be silenced. Maybe one day we can just comfortably be whoever and whatever we are.

LANDMINES
By Marie

My history is full of landmines in the form of memories. I try to step around them while still telling my story. It is disorienting. Calculating the time and comparing where I was to where I am makes me realize how much has happened and how far I've come, but my memories still feel fresh to the point of rawness. If I dwell on the details too long, it feels as if I will be blown apart. I still don't understand how I survived the past. All I know is that I did. I'm here. I'm queer. I'm gloriously alive.

If I am anything, I am a child of America's culture wars, raised on hardcore right-wing rhetoric, the basic premise of which was that America needed to turn back to a better time and back to (Old Testament) God.

My Catholic parents left their parish church when a new priest started using gender-neutral terms for God, and Vacation Bible School materials mentioned women as ministers. We ended up at a church sixty miles away that still had a Latin Mass, where women only wore ankle-length dresses and skirts, and still wore lace veils inside the church. This was the church I grew up in.

It's no secret that the mainstream Catholic Church has a complicated relationship with sexuality, especially when it comes to anything outside of Church-sanctioned marriage between a man and a woman. At my church, the relationship was downright toxic. There was always literature left around about the evil gay agenda destroying America and the belief that sodomy should stay illegal. In my family, it was even more personal. My father wanted to ban *The Lord of The Rings* movies after finding out one of the actors was gay. For a while, my mother hated *Finding Nemo* after discovering that a lesbian did the voice acting for Dory.

As part of this environment, I was homeschooled from kindergarten till I was eighteen, when I dropped out of my junior year to go to college. There was very little access to alternate viewpoints. It's one thing to hear bigoted sermons from the pulpit on Sunday morning. It's a totally different situation when you hear the same judgments 24/7/365 from everyone around you, right down to your textbooks and even your friends.

I spouted the same viewpoints, as well. I will never be able to forgive my fifteen-year-old self for rejecting a friend who had started to become gay friendly. She has since forgiven me and is my best friend now, but forgiving myself is harder. At least now I can understand why I acted that way, and realize that I am no longer that person.

Predictably, all of these experiences caused problems for me as a teenager when I started to realize that I wasn't just attracted to men. Until I was eighteen, all of my explicitly sexual feelings were repressed. I had crushes on boys, and sometimes even thought I was in love, but it was all very chaste. I didn't even have my first kiss until New Year's Eve 2005, by which time I was well over eighteen. After that night, it was like a wall had been smashed down, and I could no longer repress my feelings.

Not long after, I found myself reacting to women as well. Jesus, Mary, and Joseph. It hit me like a sledgehammer, if sledgehammers could be made of pure Catholic guilt and shame. If I'm being honest, there had been crushes on women before, but I had been deep, deep in denial. Suddenly, I couldn't hide from the truth anymore.

It's not like I didn't have other things to deal with. I'd had years of chronic, untreated depression and anxiety, a then-recent stint in a psychiatric hospital for suicidal urges, an addiction to cutting myself, a nasty case of bulimia, doubts about my faith, and strained relationships with the parents I still lived with. My attraction to women became another reason to hate myself. Once again, I wanted to die.

Landmines

At the same time, this revelation came at a point where my mental state was generally on an upswing. I was finally getting help for my issues, and had a wonderful therapist. Thanks to her and a new psychiatric medication, I was starting to think in new ways. Maybe, just maybe, there were alternatives to self-hatred. Maybe. Still, I was a good Catholic girl and I didn't know how to deal with what I was feeling. It wasn't going away.

"I'm going to go to see Father _____ and try to get the courage to talk to him about me thinking I'm bi. It's hard to deal with. Just knowing how my parents would reject me and be horrified, if they knew. Same-sex attraction sometimes seems worse than murder in this circle. What is wrong with me? Why can't I just be fucking SEMI-NORMAL?"

That was part of an email I sent to my then-best friend (also my first kiss). He then came out to me as bi. I didn't have a negative reaction to him; it even made me feel a little better about myself, but not much. I loved and accepted him, but I couldn't love or accept myself.

The priest was someone that my mother disliked because she thought he was too liberal. That's why I picked him. I was hoping I could find some sort of loophole. I knew exactly what the Church taught. I'd read the *Catechism* many times. Same-sex attraction was not to be acted on, and was inherently disordered and unnatural. Totally against natural law and God's plan for human sexuality. Still, I knew that there were Catholics who saw things differently. I'd grown up hearing about "Cafeteria Catholics" who didn't adhere to all of the official dogma.

Seeing Father _____ went as well as could be expected. So—laughable, cringeworthy, and scarring. Par for the course. I don't know exactly what I thought he would say, but after I tried to tell him what was going on, it was clear that I wasn't going to get the response I was hoping for. Father's opinion was that I was just vulnerable and overly sheltered, and thus reacting to anything sexual I came across. He didn't think I was a lesbian, but then, neither did I. I guess he didn't believe in bisexuality, because he totally ignored the concept even though it was the word I used.

His advice? Lose twenty pounds to be more attractive to men, and stay away from women who played softball. So much for the liberalism I was warned about. To be fair to him, he could have been a lot worse. He even meant well, in a dismissive and patronizing way. But nine years later, I wish I'd told him to go fuck himself. I wish I had been able to stand up for myself in some sort of way, but I couldn't. At least I got a story out of it that I can tell for laughs, and I've definitely made use of it. Still, it stings a little, and at the time it was devastating.

You could say that meeting was the beginning of the end of my Catholic faith. For me, there would be no loophole. No matter what the priest said, I knew my feelings were real and not going away. I was and am bisexual. In the end his dismissal was irrelevant, but at the same time it's been a long journey to self-acceptance. I couldn't easily shake off everything I had been taught since birth. Stepping inside a church became unbearable. Every Mass or Act of Confession came with crying fits and panic attacks.

Roughly a year after meeting with Father _____, I married a man in the Church. Three months later, I took a "break" from religion. I just could not take it anymore. It wasn't so much a decision as it was the reaching of a breaking point. I'd had my fill of self-flagellation.

After taking a few thousand steps back, the Catholic dogma didn't make sense to me anymore and I realized I wasn't going back. It wasn't even so much about accepting myself as it was a refusal to view others that I loved as hopelessly flawed because of their same-sex attraction. That just happened to apply to me as well. Once I started seeing holes in what I'd been taught, my faith in Catholicism and Christianity crumbled.

Leaving the church didn't mean leaving behind the guilt. It just eased it. At twenty-six, I've only just begun to explore my sexuality. Until the past year of my life, I had only slept with one person ever: the man I married. After six years, the marriage is over, and its end has also taken away some of the guilt and given me more freedom. So where do I go now, with no husband or Church? Up and up. Freedom is an amazing thing.

It has been a slow, painful process, but the more open I am, and the more I choose to be around accepting people, the more at peace I become with myself and all aspects of myself. I can't say I'll never cut myself again or never want to die, but every day I step closer to loving and accepting myself. Life isn't perfect, but it's far better than I ever thought it could have been when I was a suicidal, self-destructive conflicted teen.

I have never been able to go back to Christianity. I identify as an Eclectic Pagan now, and much to my surprise, I have found a home in my local Pagan community. It is my own little community of misfits, and I love them all dearly. Of course, I also have my Goddess and God and personal spiritual practices, which have helped me to heal in innumerable ways.

I have two young children now, and I try my best to raise them in a way that accepts them and teaches them self-acceptance. I hope they will grow up with the confidence I am still trying to gain. I want them to love themselves no matter what. Just as importantly, I want them to accept and love the people they come across in their lives.

When I look back over these words that I have written, and think about the path I've taken through life, one thing sticks out to me. I don't think it's widely understood just how integral sexual orientation is to identity. It's certainly taken me a long time to understand that. It's not just a matter of what people do behind closed bedroom doors. For me, it's not something I can compartmentalize that way. I want to be able to hold hands with a woman in public. I want to be able to mention a significant other and not have anyone bat an eye at the person's sex. I want to have the option to marry a woman and have my love be recognized and respected. I don't want to hide. I'm done with hiding and the dishonesty inherent to it. Hopefully, sharing my story means moving one step closer to a life lived with openness and integrity.

LIFE, TAKE 2
By Courgette

A few months ago, I marched in a Pride parade. I wore cute boots and danced to "Girls Just Wanna Have Fun," rainbow feather boa flapping in the breeze. I keep dutifully up to date on LGBTQ news and post important or happy or heartbreaking stories on Facebook without fear of bigoted responses. My parents have a Human Rights Campaign sticker on their car. Whenever a celebrity comes out, especially a female one, my coworker is always excited to talk to me about it. I can text my friends about my crushes, recruiting them to help with the "does-she-date-women" detective work. But dating isn't as high a priority as sitting in my quiet, cozy living room with a book, indulging in my introversion.

This is my life, but only the surface. The truth is, I have this freedom because two years ago I broke my husband's heart.

I can't give you the whole story—not even a condensed version. It's not that I can't recall, because I can. I remember each fight. I remember each time I had to leave the room to not break down in front of my daughter. I remember thinking I could fix it, and I remember the moment when I realized I couldn't. I remember every painful thing I said, and the way I had to force each word out of my mouth, already bracing myself for his tears. I remember the way I started to disassociate, because being present in those

Life, Take 2

moments was more than I could take. I couldn't form the words and feel them too.

So, I do remember. But I can't write it. I can't even think about it for more than a few moments at a time. Even now, I'm writing in vignettes. And while these sentences are true, they are also safe. They allow me to keep my distance, recalling without reliving.

On National Coming Out Day, I came out on Facebook. Everyone I actually interact with knew already, but they all cheered and liked the post and congratulated me. I thought all day long about whether I deserved to be congratulated, considering the pain I'd caused. And I wondered how my husband felt upon seeing those comments.

I don't know any coming out stories like mine. Maybe if I did, I would feel more authentic in some way, less lonely, less like the bad guy. Maybe I'd be able to reconcile the person I was with the person I am. Maybe I could understand—or, if not understand, accept—how I could be so happy, so in love, and then suddenly … not, without any tangible changes occurring.

That's the key difference between my story and the others I hear. I was happy—really happy. I was in love with the same man for twelve years. There was no closet. There was no denial. There was no conscious deception. I knew I was queer, I just didn't think I was *that* queer.

Now, I see it all reframed. I can look at my life with 20/20 hindsight, and see all the things I should have seen: all the mountains I disguised as molehills, the crushes I never acknowledged, the disinterest I chalked up to low libido. It's amazing what we can ignore when we put our minds to it. But there was joy, too, and it's more painful to remember the joy than the sadness. It feels like something was ripped away from me, like being violently awoken from a good dream.

A few weeks after I came out to my parents, my mom asked, "Are you really bi, or did you just say that to soften the blow?" I'm not sure how bisexuality could soften any part of losing her son-in-law and watching her daughter painfully dismantle her life, but she's right that I don't know how to identify. Calling myself a lesbian feels like a lie, not only because I've never dated women or slept with women, but also because it erases all the happy years I spent with my husband. From that perspective, bi seems closer to the truth; but still not quite right, as I have no intention of dating men after this. Becoming educated about transgender issues complicates things even further. Amid a more sophisticated definition of gender, what does being attracted to women even mean? More and more, I am grateful for the vagueness of the word "queer."

So, where does this leave me? Am I better off than I was? People talk about "living authentically" like they're throwing all the windows open to let in the sun. Maybe someday I'll be able to bask in my decision. For now, the light hurts my eyes and illuminates the neglected, messy corners of the room.

I AM MORE THAN MY SEXUAL ORIENTATION
By Beth Desmontagnes

When I turned nineteen, I had my first sexual encounter with a woman. That was when I realized I was bisexual. I came out to my mother, my sister, and a few close friends. One of those close friends was my very first childhood friend, so I did not hesitate to call her and tell her "I'm bisexual," to which she replied "Of course you are. I've always known that." I was so happy to know that after fifteen years of friendship we had grown close enough for her to see who I truly was, even before I myself had been able to see it.

I had moved away for college and my friend was going to visit for the first time since I had come out to her. I wasn't nervous in the slightest; I was just excited to see my old friend. It was the hottest Canada Day that I can remember. It was humid and the A/C unit in my apartment was not very efficient. I helped my friend bring her luggage in and after a quick hello and a hug, she proceeded to strip down to her underwear. I understood it was very hot at my place, but I was taken aback nonetheless. It's not like I hadn't seen her naked before, and her exposed skin did not make me uncomfortable, but I found her behavior strange and I questioned her intentions.

Is she testing me to see if I am attracted to her? Is she trying to make me see her in a sexual way? I know she is straight, but does she want me to want her? I could not tell so I tried not to read into it too much, although the whole incident left me with an uneasy feeling. We had been friends since we were four years old. She was practically my sister. I love her but I could never be attracted to her in a sexual or romantic way.

I let it slide.

Time passed and we kept in touch, but we weren't as close as we used to be. I decided to go visit her and her fiancé. We went out on the town with a few other friends from high school. As the night progressed she drank a little too much and she was definitely louder than usual. I was standing at the bar with her soon-to-be husband when she swooped in and dragged both of us off to the dance floor. She was grinding up on him and though his face said, "I haven't been drinking enough to dance like this," he humoured her and put his hands on her hips. To make light of the situation, I decided to join in. I turned my butt to her and gyrated my hips a little bit, sandwiching her in the middle.

I was laughing until I felt her hands creep up from behind me and grab my breasts. I removed her hands and turned around sharply. She then lunged forward in an attempt to kiss me. I recoiled and her fiancé had to hold her back while she continued to push towards me, puckering her lips.

"What are you doing? Stop!" I told her.

That was when she screamed out, "What? It's fine! You like girls anyway!"

I was mortified. Not only did she out me to the entire bar and sexually assault me in front of her fiancé, but she legitimately thought that because I was bisexual I was attracted to all women.

This took place years ago but it still hurts me for so many reasons. For one, my sexual orientation is *mine*. I am the person who decides when, how and to whom I come out. A true friend and ally would see me as a person, not as a fetish to be paraded around in order to make their own life more interesting and exciting. Also, the fact that I identify as bisexual does not mean I am attracted to everyone, nor does it mean that everyone is entitled to my body. I am attracted to some women, not all women. Even the women to whom I am attracted to need my consent before initiating any kind of sexual contact with me. As a bisexual woman, I do not exist as a sexual object ready and available for you at any time. If it is wrong for a man to grope me in public, the fact that you are a woman and I am bisexual does not somehow make your actions acceptable.

As a pansexual woman who often identifies as bisexual (because most of the time I do not feel like explaining myself), I mostly struggle with invisibility. Although I am queer, my gender performance is mostly femme. I happen to have a vagina and I enjoy wearing makeup and dresses, so most of the time I pass as a cis gender straight woman. In these instances an important part of me is rendered invisible; it is as though I am only being partially seen.

The story I have shared with you is a story about invisibility, though it is not necessarily about bisexual erasure. When I came out to my friend, it was all *but* my bisexuality that was erased. All she saw was my sexual orientation, but I am so much more than that. I enjoy reading, writing, and cooking. I like to think I have a good sense of humour. I prefer dogs to cats. I care for my friends and my family members. There are a million things that make me who I am, and my sexual orientation is only one of them.

To only see me as a person who is attracted to men and women (and everything in between) is to deny me my person hood. I wish that for once my bisexuality could be visible and acknowledged without without simultaneously erasing the rest of who I am. When I first came out to my friend, I was happy because I thought she saw who I truly was. It seems I was mistaken.

TO BE, OR NOT TO BE
By Danielle Hamilton

To be, or not to be, that is the question. As a child, I always paid more attention to the girls. I stared a little longer than others did. At that age, how do you even begin to tell anyone about it? As I grew up, my parents were accepting of everyone except me, it seemed. Thank God at this point I hadn't had a real crush, though I had my share of boyfriends and enjoyed the attention. I knew myself outright before anyone else did, and I also knew that one day I'd have to show my true self.

And then I met her. She was so beautiful, and I would be so mean to her. I even joined an after-school drama class to just look at her. Once summer commenced after that school year, I was staying the night at a friend's house and she invited another girl over. And what do you know—it was her. After our mutual friend fell asleep, we sat together writing notes to each other in a notebook all night long. Her every word was my encore to continue.

We became inseparable.

Then it was that dreaded time: the time to tell someone, so I told my best friend, who was totally accepting. The next school year started again soon after, and though I never broadcasted it, my inclinations were a known thing. I heard my fair share of "How?" and "Why?" I came to realize there was not an explanation beyond this fact: you are forever who you are.

But not everyone understands that. Ignorance is bliss, I guess.

I made it official on MySpace (back when people still had that). Soon my parents found out and told me they thought I was disgusting and wrong—which is hard to hear. I simply asked, "Why can't you accept me for who I am?" They replied, "Because who you are is wrong." My parents still think it's a phase, still to this day, which just goes to show that there will always be someone who objects to who you are.

Obviously, I'm not going to say this path was all easy. However, here is what I've learned in the process, time and time again: you're most comfortable when you accept yourself, because you will forever be who you are and deep down, nothing can change that.

IT SHOULDN'T HAVE TO BE A SECRET
By Grace Carroll

I'M GOING TO WRITE THIS ANONYMOUSLY because I have not come out—nor do I see myself doing so with my family the way they are right now. However, the people who matter—they know. That means you. That also means my husband.

I guess the long and short of my story is this: I don't fit into a category. I'm not straight but I'm not "one way" either. I've come to understand that I'm probably bisexual, but I happen to have a soul mate who is male, therefore making our relationship heterosexual. If I fell in love with another girl and made a life with her, I would not be viewed as such, but seeing as the love of my life is a man, it's easy to hide.

I've always been attracted to both genders, and always knew of sexuality and what it meant. I always thought I would grow up to marry a prince, and be his princess. But as I grew older, it wasn't so clear. While I had many close friends of both genders, I also found myself attracted to people of both genders. As I'm writing this, I'm getting a lump in my throat because I have kept this secret for twenty-four years. It shouldn't have needed to be kept secret.

I write to tell others they're not alone. No matter how old you are, no matter how you were raised—you're not alone. Sometimes you're just born not fitting into a type or category, and it's hard to admit that because it makes people generally uncomfortable. I mean, if you don't know "what" you are, how are others to interpret that? With confusion? As a lack of faith, if you're of a fundamentalist background like me—or worse, as spiritual warfare? As Satan trying to "win you over" by putting "unholy" feelings deep within your soul?

I'm still discovering who I am spiritually, mentally, emotionally, and even sexually. It shouldn't have taken me a quarter of a century to do so—but there it is. Thanks for letting me write a little something on this topic. It means a lot that I can share this with others who may be feeling the same way.

SO TELL ME ABOUT YOUR CHILDHOOD: HOW THERAPY SAVED MY SEXUALITY AND SENSE OF SELF
By Johnnie Stevens

For the longest time, I listened to the propaganda. You know the kind.

"You have to choose one side."

"You just can't pick, and that's why you're bi."

And, as I'm sure many bi or pansexuals know, you get it from both sides. Both the straight and gay people had me fooled: sexuality was a binary. They had me convinced I was only bisexual so that I could be straight for my highly fundamentalist Christian parents and gay for my friends. I could fit in at poetry slams and at church. They said I was "choosing the coward's way." I was "afraid to lose friends and come out."

As a child who discovered masturbation very early, I was damned from both ends. Sexuality wasn't discussed in my home, let alone alternate sexuality. Whether I touched myself to the idea of a man or a woman, GI Joe or Barbie, the fact remained: I was touching myself, and that, in and of itself, was wrong. At age seven, when I kissed a girl on the playground, I was told simply not to do it again—but never why not. I don't remember what reason my parents gave, but I assumed it was because it was a sexual act, not because I was a girl and had kissed a girl. I played dress-up with friends and always wanted to be the boyfriend. At around age ten, I had one girl friend stop coming over because "it was getting weird, playing pretend like that."

At fourteen, the issue of sexuality and my confusion became worse as some of my friends started coming out. Where did this leave me? What was I? Was I easily definable? Clearly not, as I had a huge crush on a boy from Ceramics one year, and the next, a girl in Earth Science.

My family moved across the country the year I turned fifteen. With that new start, I could be who I wanted; I could leave behind my past. But I found myself falling into similar ruts. Though I could now identify as bisexual at school, I did so rarely and, only among a few friends, because I feared the similar sense of rejection and the labels of "coward" or "doormat." Kids at my new school were much less conservative and sex was suddenly a huge topic. I started the process of defining my sexuality, but growth and exploration were stunted by the fear of condemnation from ingrained religious beliefs and rejection from others.

The summer after my senior year, I broke up with a boy that I had been very serious with in high school. Though we were never very physical, he had been a good friend. I went on a trip back to my hometown and visited a bunch of old friends, including a woman who had come out right after I had moved away. She and I hung out, and that night, we got intimate. It was my first time having anything near sex, let alone with a woman. She was lovely and kind. The evening was fun, and I thought we were both happy with that. But it turned out my partner wasn't: she was looking for a deeper connection, something I was unable to provide from my place of brokenness. I had just ended a relationship with someone else, and I was hurt, numbed. I wasn't really looking for serious relationships or anything committed. I didn't verbalize this, but neither did my female partner verbalize her desire for something serious. As such, our very good friendship crumbled the next morning after she became aware of our mutual unmet expectations. I viewed it as singularly my fault, mostly because she did, as well. I was the slut. I was the one who had "tricked her."

This experience, combined with being used for several women's "try out" periods during my freshman year of college, made me think that maybe—maybe—women were just a sexual fascination. Something I could write off as "a phase." Up until a year ago, I was content to have that be that, and just forget the whole damn thing. In my mind, faking straight was easier than anything else. I would masturbate mostly to women or whatever man I may have been with at the time, and feel guilty either way about touching myself. I would spend the rest of the day thinking everyone else could smell the shameful scent of my sex on my fingers.

I dated one man throughout the rest of college. He and I became very serious, even talking about marriage and kids. The rest of college went pretty well. I made straight A's my senior year. I landed an excellent internship. I was able to push religious guilt to the back of my mind—which was not at all like actually confronting the guilt and shame. I didn't go to church because I didn't want to. In retrospect, I could have seen that as a sign.

Then graduation came, along with that gut-wrenching "What now?" feeling. I moved back home with my parents after graduation, and began to regress in my sense of freedom. I stopped hanging out with my boyfriend later at night, because it made my parents uncomfortable. I started to lie to them about sex. I started to feel shameful in said sexual encounters with my boyfriend. I went to church with my parents every Sunday. I was hurting, but masked that hurt with the assumption that the pain was just due to missing college and people my own age.

I began to attend my own church because my parents' church was too conservative. They were somewhat understanding, but as my older sister put it, it was also a bit of an ordeal. "This means you're taking your faith seriously," she asserted. I didn't know if that was true; I just think I wanted friends. As an attempt to make more friends who I thought might listen or understand, I attended a twenty-something group. But they were superficial, quick-fix Christians. Whenever I would talk about my problems with my parents, boyfriend, or job, they'd provide the "God will heal all," kind of advice. It felt like a Band-aid that was stuck on everything. When they found out my boyfriend was an atheist, they told me the relationship "wasn't good for me," "impossible to make work," and that I should "just stop hurting myself." I didn't feel hurt by the relationship. I felt hurt, confused, and alone by not knowing where I stood. My boyfriend and I started fighting more about increasingly stupid things. I stopped hearing my own desires and was overwhelmed by the desire to just please everyone else. Once more, the messages and feelings of shame surrounded my love and sexuality; my lover, and the one I chose, was not good enough, and by association, neither was I.

After a while, I felt myself breaking under pressure. I couldn't hear my own voice anymore, and in a failed attempt to make everyone else happy, my boyfriend and I broke up. I sobbed for two days straight. Heartbroken, I entered therapy, which was completely terrifying. "Good girls don't need therapy," was the lie I told myself. I had lost everything; the world had unraveled at my feet. But my therapist was wonderful. She saw before I did what had really been occurring: the theme of my life was a betrayal of self. In an attempt to please everyone, I had lost my own desires, my own voice, my own dreams.

When I came out to my therapist, I cried the entire session. I told her I felt wrong and dirty and would just rather avoid the topic. I was swiftly told that meant it was exactly what we needed to be talking about. And so we talked about it . . . for the next three weeks. My therapist pointed out that every time I talked about sexual thoughts, about either men or women, I held my head down. That made me start to cry. How had I become so ashamed of something so natural? In an eerie way, just having her point that out helped me realize how much I had shrouded my sexuality in shame and "badness." Due to her prompting, I began to speak frankly about sex, almost as a dare. Sometimes, in an attempt to compensate for the years of non-discussion, we over-discussed sexuality, sexual thoughts, and sexual behaviors. But for the first time in my life, I wasn't cringing at the word "vagina." I started to see women as multidimensional again, to feel validity in my desire for them, and to not just feel shame. I began to accept my sexual thoughts, desires, and actions.

Over the next year, I learned the power of myself and of my voice. I came out to my counselor and to my best Christian friend (both times, I was met with the kindest love—I know I am more than lucky in this). I got back together with my boyfriend. I moved in with the most loving woman I know, who also happens to be an atheist. I stopped going to church, coming to peace with the idea that God (and the way I experience God) is an entity that does not fit in the preconceived, conservative boundaries that I previously experienced.

After a year and a half of therapy, and currently one month out of therapy standing on my own two feet, I'm joyful in my life. My boyfriend and I are monogamous, and he's not threatened by the fact that I identify as pansexual. I am loyal to him, but no longer think in black-and-white terms about my sexuality. The people I am out with have loving, genuine conversations with me about sexuality: mine, their own, and in general.

    I have never felt more content in my beliefs. While I'm not out to my family, the therapeutic process has organically begun some deeper conversations about God, hurt, and love. Maybe I'll come out to my parents some day, but the point is, I don't any longer feel like I'm lying to them or to anyone else—including myself. I've found peace within my sexuality, my relationship, and myself. There are still times I feel moments of shame and hurt, but overall, I just feel like myself: this wonderful, paradoxical person, who will never again try to fit herself into a box.

MOTHER OF PEARL
By Sophie Unruh

When I was quite young, I learned a trick. I learned to dream while I was still awake.

I dreamed I lay in a shallow pool. The water streamed away and around me. A slender stream was falling into the pool from over a ledge. The sky shone through the trees like mother of pearl.

I lay in the water, waiting.

A freshwater clam was resting, closed, under the waterfall. In the quiet that I was feeding it, the began to unlock. It's shell opened. Sitting inside was a pearl.

Because I had gotten the clam to open, the pearl was mine. And it wasn't just a pretty bead. It was whole and perfect, and for someone gifted with my powers, it was a gateway to time and space and everything outside them as well.

* * *

She laid her piece down. She seemed bored, at first, but her excitement at figuring out the game was welling up and molting the boredom. This was the first time she'd played Go. I would be lucky to win against her even this once.

We didn't know each other very well. She was breaking up with one of my guy friends. Before that, she had broken up with a future that she had trained for all her childhood.

I had just broken up with the first boy who'd ever liked me—who I felt nothing for. And I'd emotionally disentangled myself from the first boy I had ever fallen for—who felt nothing for me. I had fallen for him all the way. I was much older than what seemed to be normal for such experiences. Getting over them was the hardest thing I'd yet done.

When her breakup was over, we kept hanging out. We went to church together. Shortly thereafter, I moved and we fell out of touch.

She was brilliant with math and language. She could see the patterns while most people were still trying to see what the pieces were. That was why she was giving me a run for my money during her first game of Go, when I had introduced her to the game in the first place.

I myself played Go because the pieces and shapes were called Stars and Dragons and Liberties. I assume my strategies were poetic. They certainly didn't win me anything.

I couldn't understand why the world kept lighting up around her. Why my heart kept moving so strangely.

* * *

In the dream world, I was a sorcerer. I could tie a person up with a daisy chain and it would hold them like iron. I could plunge a dagger into a footprint and the entire trail would light up with fire, all the way to the feet that were setting prints in the soil.

It was a dangerous world. Exciting and beautiful, but dangerous.

If someone caught a sorcerer, they would drown that sorcerer. The dying of any kind have a moment of truth as they slip out of the world. The unlucky sorcerer would sink, heart pounding, tongue stopped with water—and the living would be spared from hearing those particular truths.

* * *

Mother Of Pearl

Sitting in town one day and eating lunch outside, I idly watched the people walking by across the street.

A woman walked past. She was a little chubby, wearing bright colors and a solidly-filled halter top. Her hair was tied up in a bandana and spilling in black curls out the back.

I gasped. My whole body was suddenly glowing.

I had grown up homeschooled out in the country. Somewhere in my mother's eight pregnancies, I had heard some of the mechanical details of sex that were necessary for reproduction. Television (when we had a set) was monitored. We had very few neighbors, no internet, and few interactions with people who weren't close relatives.

My mom talked in a sad voice about my one gay uncle. There was a distant lesbian relative whom she called Aunt Sewer.

Our family was more liberal than some families we knew. Far more liberal than some others we knew of.

If we weren't going anywhere, we girls wore sleeveless shirts. We hid that indiscretion from some of our acquaintances.

I had wordlessly figured that feeling out for myself. It was . . . sexual. It was desire. I had it when I thought of certain boys. I had it when I thought of pain. I could no longer pretend that I didn't have it for girls, too.

Growing up, I had heard you were supposed to put out your eyes rather than look with lust. Rather than look with desire.

She walked on by.

* * *

In some forms of the dream, I lived in a tower with one other girl: my sister. We lived there alone.

I could do magic. She could fight. I had soft clothes, and she had brown leather and a sword. She laughed and teased people when she fought them. I walked in the forest and barely talked to anyone.

We had a friend who came and went, not trapped by taking care of a tower like we were.

He was a sorcerer like me. Quick on his feet and quick with his words, he didn't fight. He charmed his way out of difficulties. He laughed too.

In other forms of the dream, I went off with him instead. Sometimes he would get caught and I would save him. Sometimes I would get caught and he would save me.

Always, there was some grand quest. What it was eludes me now—just a quest like they always were. We went. Either I went with him and she came along too, or I went with her and he came along as well.

Every form of the dream made me happy. I loved them.

* * *

Dreams tend to get old and frail as time passes. Even waking dreams can die. As I got older, this happened to me. Though I don't use my trick nearly as much as I did when I was young, it wasn't my dream world that died.

It was my mother's world that died, the world that appeared to have been her personal fantasy of religion and God and a woman's place in life—pregnant and in the kitchen. It was the dream with which she had organized her life and ours.

It didn't die for her. It didn't die for her other children. It died for me.

I would have been willing to live by it at whatever cost to myself, whatever I had to hide, as long as I thought it was real. But it simply wasn't. It wasn't true. It is, perhaps, a story for another time.

Without that, I can't keep my entire life in my head anymore. It simply doesn't fit. It spills out onto the trail of footprints I've left behind me. The soil transmutes it. The imaginary flowers grow up on soft stems, real and sturdy as iron, binding me to things I can't escape any longer.

I walk out in the dust and under the sun. I know myself better now. Between the dust and the clouds, the sky has become a clam shell holding one freshwater pearl. The years of walking in two worlds are ending.

Strange as it may sound for someone who swings all the ways I do, for as far as I can scry into my future, I will be living in one world—only one world.

Whoever else happens to be in it, it will be my world.

PART THREE:
REFLECTION AND ANALYISIS

BISEXUALITY IN SOCIETY AND CULTURE

THROUGH AN INTERPLAY OF SOCIAL FORCES and the criminal legal system, gender and sexuality undergo constant social and literal policing.[1] In order to keep social circles "pure" and reinforce current power structures, people who deviate from cishet norms face censure, marginalization, and prejudice.

In the typical Western cishet narrative, there are only the male and female genders, and these genders are determined by examining genitalia. Using an outdated measurement left over from ancient history, men retain dominance and authority while women find value in marriage and childbearing. Through legal records of marriage, legitimate offspring, and inheritance, wealth and power are retained by a few families. This system also favors the white and wealthy over people of color, poor people, and the working classes. People in the middle class are often deeply invested in this system because although it is not primarily set up to benefit them, they believe it can enable them to join the hyper-privileged upper classes. Concurrently, by turning their frustration and anger toward those even less

---

1 For an excellent examination of the oppression faced by queer people in the hands of the criminal legal system, read Joey L Moguel, Andrea J. Ritchie, and Kay Whitlock, *Queer (In)Justice: The Criminalization of LGBT People in the United States* (Boston, MA: Beacon Press, 2011).

privileged than themselves, people in the lower classes will sometimes shore up the very system that oppresses them.

As stated earlier, cishet norms are founded upon a system of patriarchal dominance. Those invested in such a power-hungry structure cannot simply live and let live; our entire culture must conform or else the system of dominance loses its power. Self-perpetuation of ideology only happens when people believe there is no other reasonable option, and so to the cishet patriarchal system, a happy queer is an enormous threat. The moment someone steps outside of gender norms, they individually render the entire system of dominance and privilege invalid. And when a person steps outside of heterosexuality, they likewise render this system impossible.

Although certain non-heterosexual partnerships are now smiled upon by the dominant system, only those that closely align with cishet norms are given such approval. Even liberal folks, many of whom identify as "progressive," often prefer monogamous gay or lesbian couples who appear to mimic heterosexual couples. What little respect is afforded to transgender people is typically reserved for those who pass as cisgender. Only by forfeiting as much of our queerness as possible are queer people allowed to enter into the cishet systems of privilege and power. If a brave individual or group stands up to suggest that perhaps we queer folk are not, or should not be, interested in or confined by the stipulations of entering into power and privilege, they are all too often mocked, marginalized, and repressed. The system of dominance must remain total.

As bisexuals, not only do we face general pressure to conform as closely as possible to cishet romantic and relational narratives, we also face pressure to perform our queerness according to the stereotypes provided through a deluge of misinformation about our sexuality. Particularly within the mainstream media, our existence is regularly erased or reduced to a single letter by politicians and news anchors who use the catch-all term "LGBT" in their discussions of the (largely cis) gay movement.

The media consistently invalidates bisexual celebrities, speaking of them as though as they are simply switching between being gay and being straight, as though their sexuality changes based on their partner. When the person in question must continually explain bisexuality in each and every interview they give, they are still mislabeled and misrepresented. The dominant structures in our society require that each person surrender their gender and sexuality. Who you are, and who you love, and how you structure your relationships—these things do not belong to you. They must be examined and controlled by others, by systems meant to destroy or de-fang the subversive potential of sexual autonomy. In dealing with people who try to fit sexuality into a mold created by someone else, bisexuals must insist that our sexuality is all our own. Yet again we find ourselves at the forefront of a disruptive argument. We insist that each person hold full ownership of their own gender and sexuality, and thus we confront and contradict the prurient, controlling culture that is intent on enforcing cishet norms.

Many popular interpretations of bisexuality center on cishet men. As Shiri Eisner points out in *Bi: Notes for a Bisexual Revolution*, "for bisexual women the presumption is that we're really straight, while bisexual men are often presumed to [actually] be . . . gay. This suggests a presumption that everyone is really into men—a phallocentric notion testifying to this stereotype's basic reliance on sexism."[2]

When bisexuality is acknowledged as real, the cishet male gaze centers upon itself, appropriating female bisexuality for its own pleasure and expecting women (or feminine-presenting people) to exaggeratedly perform their sexuality. A man may automatically reduce "bisexual" to a signifier that a woman is interested in a female-female-male threesome, or that she will make out with another girl for the man's enjoyment but afterwards choose to go to bed with only him. He may feel secure enough to mock her as a "barsexual" or as "bicurious," because he does not believe it possible that she would choose a female partner over his phallus. This feeling of entitlement to pleasure can quickly turn to lashing out and abuse when rejection, infidelity, or exercise of personal autonomy is suspected.

Alternatively, a woman may express same-sex desire as part of a "one of the guys" performance of, or striving for, masculinity or masculine approval. (It is noteworthy that this performance is never inverted; for men to express same-sex desire in a bid to gain the approval of women is not seen, by cishet norms, to be socially profitable.) There is no clear way to know how much female same-sex expression of desire is due to the overbearing presence of an objectifying, patriarchal culture that glorifies masculine possession of women. We may not be able to tell whether a woman is seeking to access

---

2 Eisner, *Bi*, 39.

the privilege, power, and the approval of masculinity by expressing desire she does not feel, or whether she is using this role to express desire she does genuinely feel. Women who seek approval from patriarchal society by enacting "masculine" domination of other women can benefit from striving to unlearn patriarchy's teachings, and becoming more honest about their own desires, whether they identify as bisexual or not.

While the "one of the guys" role provides a (problematic) outlet for exploring sexuality, it is frequently used in media (particularly on television) to allow female characters a measure of masculine approval without questioning their assumed straight identity. This misshapen media representation teaches viewers to interpret female expressions of same-sex desire in ways that center on fantasies of masculine possession of women.[3] Such skewed portrayals contribute greatly to the erasure ("I know you are actually straight") and objectification ("can I join in?") of bi women.

The cishet male gaze fears and mocks male bisexuality, viewing it as a direct challenge to its own stringently-policed straightness. Many cishet men can be offended equally by the thoughts that a bisexual man might find them attractive, or that he might not. Each possibility is seen by the cishet man as an assault on his perception of his own masculinity. Bisexual men are seen as infiltrators of the cishet male brotherhood, betraying the patriarchy with their refusal to base their sexuality on possessing and exploiting women. Perhaps for this reason, male bisexuality is not publicly fetishized to the same extent as female or feminine bisexuality. However, bisexual men and masculine-presenting people are still at risk for homophobic and biphobic violence, erasure, and the vicious mockery visited upon those who do not live up to the cishet standard of "manliness."

Sometimes prejudice against bisexuals is implied, or acted out rather than spoken. But at other times, its presence is made painfully obvious as soon as the topic of bisexuality is broached. In my personal life, I have had several men openly muse to me about what it would be like to watch me have sex with another woman. One evening, in particular, some of my friends began to speculate about a male friend's sexuality. At first I was pleased that they even knew the word bisexual, and were able to understand that our

---

3   For a discussion of performance of bisexuality for cishet male pleasure in pornography, see Eisner, *Bi*, 162–174.

friend was not necessarily gay or straight. Unfortunately, the conversation quickly devolved as one man finally took over the entire conversation by loudly declaring, "He'd better not be staring at my butthole!" over and over again, automatically assuming that a man who was attracted to men must therefore be attracted to *all* men, including him.

In an atmosphere such as this, bisexuals must proclaim more emphatically than anyone else, "My sexuality is mine. It is not for others to interpret or control, nor does it exist to fuel others' sexual fantasies." Through this proclaimation, we find ourselves allied with lesbians, who also often face the expectation that they will "perform" for cishet men. We find ourselves allied with trans and genderqueer people, who must constantly say to cis people, "My gender and my genitals are mine; they are not open for dissection by your curious gaze." Trans people face far greater violation, at much higher rates, at the hands of cis people who believe they are entitled to an explanation of intimate details of trans people's transitions, genitals, and sex lives. To enrich allyship with fellow bisexuals who are trans, and with non-bi trans people, cis bisexuals should draw from their personal experiences of inappropriately intimate queries and attempts at cishet control.

Despite all this violation, erasure and misunderstanding of bisexuality may, for some, seem to be minor problems when compared to physical and sexual violence. Misrepresentation and invisibility might often result in nothing worse than a little mental distress (or perhaps sore throats, as bisexuals spend the majority of their time explaining what being bi does and does not mean, that being bi is real, and that no, we aren't just doing this for attention or to fulfill somebody's threesome fantasy). However, these seemingly harmless challenges based in perceptions and ideas can lead directly to real-world harm and very serious violence.

When bi people are considered too queer for straight society, violence frequently arises at the hands of enraged partners, acquaintances, or even strangers. As William Burleson points out in *Bi America: Myths, Truths, and Struggles Of an Invisible Community*, "no 'gay basher' stops to ask exactly where someone falls on the Kinsey scale. No one is only *half*-bashed because [they are] bi."[4] Many monosexual people do not stop to think about this fact,

---

4   William E. Burleson, *Bi America: Myths, Truths, and Struggles of an Invisible Community* (Binghamton, NY: Harrington Park Press, 2005), 19.

and assume there is no particular threat of violence against bi people—after all, we can pass as straight, can't we?

Regularly, blame for the distress that comes from experiencing biphobia and living in a world that rejects bisexuals is wrongly placed on our shoulders. When this misplacement occurs, we can be subjected to conversion therapy—by even non-religious, "qualified," yet still biphobic therapists. Any therapist or mental health worker who implies that being bisexual is part of a personality disorder, or that our sexuality stems from abuse or trauma during childhood, or even that happiness can be achieved purely by "just choosing to be gay or straight," is only exacerbating our psychological distress. Such practitioners should be discredited in the same way we discredit religious conversion therapists who target gay and lesbian children to "turn them straight."

Akin to other sexual minorities who must flee from countries that violently persecute them, bisexuals who seek political asylum are often asked to "prove" their identities to a governing body that determines whether or not asylum will be granted. Often, upon failing to prove themselves (an innately difficult task), bi people are denied asylum, which leads to direct physical harm, deprivation of resources, and even death.[5]

Hypersexualization, stemming from media misrepresentation, may also be a contributing factor to disproportionately high rates of rape against bisexual women.[6] Hypersexualization leads to the assumption that a person is always ready to have sex and therefore *cannot* be raped; women of color in particular face this stigma, which is derived from historical stereotypes concocted in the minds of white men to justify the abuse of enslaved Black women. Consequently, bisexual Black women are an even more vulnerable

---

5 The case of Orashia Edwards, a bisexual man seeking asylum in the UK from Jamaica, is a current example of this kind of injustice. See Owen Duffy, "Bisexual Asylum Seeker Facing Imminent Deportation From UK to Jamaica," *The Guardian*, May 5, 2015, accessed June 20, 2015, www.theguardian.com/uk-news/2015/may/05/bisexual-jamaica-asylum-seeker-facing-imminent-deportation-from-uk

6 M.L. Walters, J. Chen, & M.J. Breiding. *The National Intimate Partner and Sexual Violence Survey (NISVS): 2010 Findings on Victimization by Sexual Orientation.* (Atlanta, GA: National Center for Injury Prevention and Control, Centers for Disease Control and Prevention, 2013).

population. This problem will be discussed in greater depth in the upcoming section.

Of course, bi erasure and misrepresentation is not just something that occurs on TV. It occurs in medical literature as well. In a survey of medical literature spanning two decades, Kaestle and Ivory found that "most of the medical literature dealing with sexual minorities either ignores bisexuals or collapses them into categories with homosexuals."[7] When doctors do not receive accurate information about how to care for bisexuals' unique healthcare needs, bisexuals receive, at best, incomplete healthcare and health information. As the San Francisco Human Rights Commission (SFHRC) report points out, the typical biphobic assumption is that "bisexual people [should] get services, information, and education from heterosexual service agencies for their 'heterosexual side' and then go to gay and/or lesbian service agencies for their 'homosexual side.'"[8] This assumption leads not only to poor healthcare for bisexuals, but also to resources being channeled primarily toward gay and lesbian organizations, as donors and government organizations operate under the notion that bi people will be comparably served by programs for gays and lesbians. When surveys about sexual minorities lump bisexuals in with lesbians and gay men, this "makes it difficult to draw any conclusions about bisexuals *and* skews the data about lesbians and gay men."[9] As pointed out later in the SFHRC report, when it comes to problems such as suicide and domestic abuse (which are both often faced at higher rates by bisexual populations), such conflation continues to lead to bisexuals being underserved while needed resources are diverted toward gays and lesbians. Thus, not only does bi erasure endanger bisexuals by cutting off important, often life-saving resources, but it also contributes to inequality and marginalization of bisexuals within the LGBT community.

Bisexual erasure, misrepresentation, hypersexualization, and disinformation are not trivial concerns. These issues can lead directly to

---

[7] Christine Elizabeth Kaestle and Adrienne Holz Ivory, "A Forgotten Sexuality: Content Analysis of Bisexuality in the Medical Literature over Two Decades," *Journal of Bisexuality* 12:1 (2012): 35, accessed August 11, 2014, doi: 10.1080/15299716.2012.645701.

[8] San Francisco Human Rights Commission, LGBT Advisory Committee, "Bisexual Invisibility: Impacts and Recommendations" (San Francisco, CA, 2011), 6.

[9] San Francisco Human Rights Commission, "Bisexual Invisibility," 3.

physical harm and deprivation, to the point of endangering bi people's lives. The psychological stress of stigma, biphobia, and erasure can cause negative consequences in the lives of bisexuals as well. When we speak about the cishet patriarchal system oppressing us, we, as bisexuals, are talking about something that is slowly, steadily killing us and urgently needs to be overthrown.

BISEXUALITY IN QUEER POLITICS AND THE CHANGING AMERICAN FAMILY

"Of course, we too will be fighting to defeat the anti-queer marriage amendments. How can we not? But we resent having to do it, and we will not allow it to distract us from our real needs: equality, justice, self-determination, and self-actualization for ALL. Just because you are not someone's significant other, does not mean you are insignificant."

— Kate and Deeg.[1]

QUEER POLITICS, BELIEVE IT OR NOT, do not begin and end with gay marriage. Mass focus on gaining same-sex marriage rights (notably different from gay marriage rights, as bisexuals' rights are simultaneously expanded when same-sex marriage is legalized) has created a taboo about questioning whether the privileges reserved for marriage should even be connected to said institution. However, money, energy, and attention are expended disproportionately on the issue of marriage rights while queer kids on the street continue to be harassed and beaten by cops, while gay, lesbian, bisexual, and particularly transgender people go without employment

---

[1] Kate and Deeg, "Marriage is Still the Opiate of the Queers," in *Against Equality: Queer Revolution Not Mere Inclusion*, ed. Ryan Conrad (Oakland, CA: AK Press, 2014), 49.

protection in many workplaces, while housing discrimination remains legal—and on and on.

The main goal of queer liberation must never be mere "safe" acceptance into society as it currently exists; it must never be simply adding ourselves to the presently privileged classes of people. All action must be undertaken with an eye toward subverting and tearing down oppressive hierarchy. The necessity of subverting oppression is precisely why bisexual activism should be centered on finding other avenues of liberation and building creative alternatives to existing structures, instead of issues of assimilation, like legal marriage and access to military service. We should be more concerned with other avenues of liberation and with creative alternatives to existing structures. We should, for instance, focus on examining the forces of poverty that offer a military career as the only way out for underprivileged youth. We should strive to feel greater solidarity with bisexuals abroad and those struggling to survive under the guns of American imperialism than we do with the United States military complex. We should be more concerned with economic justice—with ending slave labor, exploitation, and sweatshops, with restoring power to the working class—than with having an openly bisexual CEO of a multinational corporation or bank. Not everything that might be hailed by the mainstream as an "advance" for the bisexual community is actually a good thing.

At the present moment, it's fashionable for many to deride "identity politics" as a distraction from the broader struggle against capitalism, imperialism, and ecological destruction. But this rationale creates a false dichotomy. Whether discussing the disproportionate effect of climate change upon poor communities of color, or the economic disparities faced by many bisexual and transgender people at higher rates than those faced by monosexual or cis people,[2] it becomes clear that identity does indeed change perspectives on even the most vital, systemic, all-encompassing issues. No matter what we face as bisexuals (and non-monosexuals in general), we face it as ourselves. If we are asked to set our identities aside in the name of pure socialism or any other cause, we will be poorer activists and allies because

---

[2] National Center for Transgender Equality and the National Gay and Lesbian Task Force, *National Transgender Discrimination Survey: Preliminary Findings*. (Washington DC: National Gay and Lesbian Task Force, 2009).

of it. The cishet white man who cannot pay off his student loans might not think that his identity has anything to do with the financial crisis, but the Black bisexual woman whose home was just foreclosed on cannot help but understand that her identity is a part of her economic situation. If you're asked to "leave identity politics out of it," what is typically meant is, "react to this issue the way the default human (read: cishet white male) would react to it."

To build a society that is substantively different than the one we live in currently, we must first lose this assumption of the cishet white male as the "default human." Identity is only viewed as a "distraction" when a dominant group insists on perpetuating oppression against the marginalized. Meaningful revolution will only come when we embrace our identities as a whole, respect and celebrate the identities of those different from us, and use our individual unique knowledge to inform our vision of radical social change.

Discrimination against non-cisgender and non-heterosexual people is not accidental. It is not simply because we are "new" or "unusual." Queerness, although not labeled or manifesting in exactly the ways seen today, has existed throughout time and across cultures. Queer folk are not hated merely because of "the ick factor," which in and of itself seems manufactured to marginalize non-cishet identities; would anyone perceive such identities as disgusting if we did not live in a cishet-normative society? Nor can such hate be combatted only by educating others and mainstreaming our identities. No, discrimination against all who are not unerringly cishet occurs very much on purpose, and filters through many strata of society. But by radically expanding sexuality and gender, and by insisting upon acceptance as we are, instead of how we were told to be, we strike at the authority of the state. We disrupt the seemingly most sacred unit, the family, which capitalism both glorifies and exploits. We question the ability of law to dictate who we may be and who we may love. We envision a daring future in which humanity, rather than law or tradition, is allowed the autonomy to choose relationships—familial, social, sexual, and otherwise.

Non-monosexuality reveals the limitations of same-sex marriage legalization and the limited ability of the law to defend identity. Currently, it is not identity but behavior that can be sanctioned by law, yet identity can be and is still discriminated against (for example, bisexuals are explicitly mentioned in the now-overturned "Don't Ask Don't Tell").[3] Sexuality, we discover, is not equivalent to sexual activity, as non-monosexuals are placed in a legal no-man's-land based purely upon our behavior. Monogamous straight people and monogamous gay people may be legally recognized and afforded privileges by the state, but we non-monosexuals can only be recognized by masquerading as straight or gay. The law codifies the assumption that gay and straight are the only legalizable choices. As we explore what law can and cannot do, we begin to understand that fighting for legal protection and recognition of our relationships by the state cannot be the main focus of queer activism.

If marriage as a legal and religious institution has little protective power for non-monosexuals, we must ask, what is the real reason for marriage? If it is simply a commitment between people who love each other, why should certain rights be assigned to the formalization of that commitment? Should not these rights be available to all family units? As Ryan Conrad asks in *Queering Anarchism*, "What if we, as a queer and trans social justice movement, focused on achieving access to many of marriage's forbidden fruits (i.e., healthcare, freedom of movement across nation-state borders, etc.) for all people, not just citizen couples, gay, straight, or otherwise?"[4] While we work to alleviate the oppression of queer families, by broadening access to marriage for those who want or need the privileges it affords, we must also stop the agglomeration of state-given privileges for one particular type of familial partnership.

In America, the white, middle class, monogamous, cishet two-parent family is the perfect specimen of a Platonic standard against which all other families are measured. Unlike many have been led to believe, this standard is not the most natural family arrangement—nor is it an inherently bad family arrangement. However, the notion that it is the only proper family arrangement is a fiction devised for the benefit of industrial capitalism and white supremacy. At the onset of the Industrial Revolution, heterosexuality

---

3   For furhter information on bisexuality as specifically related to sexual harassment law, see Kenji Yoshino, "The Epistemic Contract of Bisexual Erasure," *Standford Law Review* 52 (2000): 353-455.

4   Ryan Conrad, "Gay Marriage and Queer Love," in *Queering Anarchism: Addressing and Understanding Power and Desire*, ed. C. B. Daring et al. (Oakland, CA: AK Press, 2012), 20.

became advertently necessary as only a cisgender, heterosexual couple could be relied upon to produce children, thereby turning the family into a (re)productive unit to perpetuate the labor force needed by capitalism.[5]

Capitalist state interest in mandating a single family type is not as brutal or overt as the control exerted over enslaved people, nor can the abuses of slavery be compared to the strictures placed on sexuality by industrial capitalism. However, in our exploration of the family under capitalism, it is important to note the differences between capitalist control of people of color and capitalist control of the white working class. If we are to grapple with oppression, if we are to subvert oppressive structures, if we are to be at all revolutionary, we must never turn a blind eye to the unique ravages that white supremacy has inflicted and continues to inflict on people of color.

At a time when enslaved Black women in America were coerced, controlled, and raped to provide more human chattel for their owners, they were valued by slave-owning whites for their ability to produce as many children as possible. But when as chattel slavery was disestablished, Black women's reproduction became societally problematized.[6] The prejudiced myth of the "welfare queen" arose in the late 20th century and is a viciously enduring stereotype to this day, though it has no basis in reality. This stereotype, and the deeming of Black children as "social problems" at their moment of birth, persists because working-class Black women living in a white supremacist capitalist society are villainized for having children who demand to be valued and dealt with as human beings—rather than as units coerced into labor. They are unlikely to be afforded the same opportunities and education as a white woman's children; their potential to create wealth for employers is thus limited. The likelihood that they will be able to escape poverty is low due to a number of mechanisms of economic and police/carceral state violence. While certain media personalities advocate

---

5   The general structure of the argument in this section is indebted the following: Eisner, *Bi*, 292–297; Ryan Conrad, ed., *Against Equality: Queer Revolution Not Mere Inclusion*, (Oakland, CA: AK Press, 2014), 15–95; Sherry Wolf, *Sexuality and Socialism: History, Politics, and Theory of LGBT Liberation* (Chicago, IL: Haymarket Books, 2009) 26–36.

6   This section on the white-supremacist, capitalist destruction of the Black family is indebted to Dorothy Roberts, *Killing the Black Body: Race, Reproduction, and the Meaning of Liberty* (New York, NY: Vintage Books, 1997).

mimicking the male-dominated, white, middle class nuclear family structure as a panacea for racism, mass incarceration is ultimately the law's solution for transforming impoverished working people, the unemployed, and those subsisting on extralegal activity into a slave-labor workforce. As a result, no matter how hard working-class Black mothers and their children work, many may remain dependent on government assistance. The blame for this incongruity is placed on the shoulders of Black mothers and their children, rather than on the institutions that continue to oppress and exploit Black people. Other women of color, especially indigenous women, face analogous discrimination in the form of forced sterilization and dangerous experimental birth control: attempts at state-administered eugenics.[7]

White people have never faced the particularly harsh nexus of control and discrimination employed against people of color. But, as a concerted society, we are all now caught up in a system (though ameliorated proportionately by race and class) where reproduction is aggressively politicized by economics, and the necessities of life are policed by the state and monetized by capitalists. As long as our society obediently functions in efficient, consumer-driven family units, producing enough children to maintain a pool of cheap, expendable labor, without demanding any "burdensome" social services, we shall never be criminalized on the basis of race or marginalized on the basis of disability—right?

It is clear that privileging the heterosexual, patriarchal, nuclear family model above all other types of families not only harms the queer community, but also functions to serve capitalism by heralding white, middle-class family arrangements as the morally superior, legally sanctioned way of having a family—while also alienating these families from community support. In the United States today, most extended family households or other non-nuclear family structures are found within communities of color. The media and politicians frequently suggest that many of the problems faced by Black Americans could be alleviated if Black Americans would adhere more strictly to a two-parent nuclear family structure. Of course, this analysis ignores the institutional violence and mass incarceration that often deprives Black families of ever-maligned Black fathers (and, more invisibly, but increasingly at similar rates, Black mothers).

---

[7] Dorothy Roberts, *Killing the Black Body.* 94–95.

Extended family units and strong community networks are vital sites of resistance against the violence, poverty, and exploitation wrought by capitalist oppressors, the police, and white supremacist laws.[8] By drawing upon these cooperative family models, queer activism around marriage and family can agitate toward an expansive goal of extending protection to all family units of whatever type or appearance.

An isolated family unit is a vital institution for the continued existence of capitalism. Glorified as the primary site for the perpetuation of values and the most important relational network in a person's life, the atomized nuclear family is often disconnected from community and possesses a weakened potential for resistance against state and capitalist power. Broader interests of the community and the possibility of forging bonds to create new, better ways of life fall by the wayside. Personal lives and interests are directed again and again back to only what is perceived as beneficial for immediate kinship groups.

Subsequently, this atomized family unit, containing the perfect consumers and the perfect citizens, produces future laborers (children) in the most efficient manner possible, by placing onto the mother the entire burden of labor that produces and nurtures the future workforce. The mother is expected to perform these tasks day and night without compensation, as she is taught that children are their own reward. The entire expense of producing and nurturing the future workforce is placed upon one or both parents (increasingly both, as wages fail to keep pace with the cost of living). In this all-too prevalent scenario, families cut off from community have a decreased chance of realizing that they are disadvantaged by capitalism—and that without them, capitalism could not exist. Therefore, rejecting the "normal" structuring of the two-parent heterosexual nuclear family can be a tool in fighting the dominance and perpetuation of capitalism. It's no

---

8   These complex familial ties have been evolving since the days of slavery, as described by George Rawick as quoted by Howard Zinn, *A People's History of the United States: 1492–Present* (New York, NY: HarperPerennial, 2005) 177–178. "The slave community acted like a generalized extended kinship system. . . the activity of the slaves in creating patterns of family life that were functionally integrative did more than merely prevent the destruction of personality. . . . It was part and parcel . . . of the social process out of which came Black pride, Black identity, Black culture, the Black community and Black rebellion in America."

wonder that the family unit remains sacrosanct, while queers who attempt to expand what family means, in practice and theory, are considered corrosive to society.

When the family is primarily viewed as a reproductive unit, same-sex couples and others who cannot reproduce are marginalized, if not actively prevented from forming their own families. The state has only recently been convinced to even recognize same-sex unions as legal. Bisexuality and other non-hetero sexualities reclaim sex as pleasure, and as a freely chosen, potentially non-procreative activity. Sex is no longer undertaken in service to the state; it is in fact blatantly, intentionally undertaken as the act of free people in service of their own desires.[9] Deviant indeed! Procreation, if proper access to medical and reproductive care is available, becomes intentional. Shockingly selfish! The state fears that unless it can turn this pleasurable, freely chosen sex, undertaken with high-caliber ethics of consent and of personal choice, back to serve itself again in some way, sex and sexuality will destabilize the whole structure of social control.

Perhaps our most unique contribution to the questioning and disruption of the nuclear family lies in the most inflammatory of all words in the gay community: *choice*. It may be true that we don't choose with whom we fall in love, but as non-monosexuals, we can potentially enter into a sexual relationship and create a family with someone of any gender. The very foundation of patriarchal control over women, as centered on family relationships, is shaken by the ability to opt out of male domination in our homes. Simply by being who we are, we are already chippings away at patriarchy. Feminism and queerness are natural allies; no matter what our gender, we can bring greater thought and intentionality to all equations, particularly when creating our own families (if we choose to do so). The

---

[9] For this thought I am indebted to Starhawk, *Dreaming the Dark: Magic, Sex, and Politics* (Boston, MA: Beacon Press, 1997), 141. "Such politics [of desire] are dangerous. They are extremely threatening to patriarchal society, because they threaten the roots of hierarchical power relationships. . . . Sexual desire for a person of one's own gender challenges the idea that the only valid purpose of sex is reproduction; it means that sexuality is valued for its own sake, for pleasure, not as a means to an end." Starhawk speaks of sex as a means of defeating the dynamics of "power-over" and instead learning "power-from-within," of learning pleasure and desire as a vital part of breaking away from the utilitarianism and consumerism of patriarchal capitalist society.

patriarchal trap—the idea that women need men and therefore cannot escape male domination, and that men require a woman to dominate—evaporates.

Unfortunately, patriarchy is not going to admit defeat so easily. The presence of men in a patriarchal society who, in the words of Eisner, find in their identity "the opportunity to step away from dominant masculinity, to refuse to be oppressors and to instead participate in the deconstruction of patriarchy"[10] is few and far between. Scarce is the occurrence of bi men who *could* choose to oppress women, but instead choose not to, "failing at performing the 'proper' standard of masculinity"[11] and using their bisexuality to betray a system that depends on male loyalty. As bi men are brushed aside, viewed as emasculated when they refuse to inhabit the typical cishet male role, bi women are taunted as "fakers" who will always come back to the "all-powerful phallus." Many heterosexual men in relationships with bi women also feel the unspoken threat to their masculine dominance given the possibility that the woman could choose to be with another woman instead; they lash out in displays of domestic violence, responding with brute force to the challenge against patriarchy that bisexual women cannot help but embody.

The capitalist cishet patriarchy has more subtly harmful ways of reinforcing the family structure, ways that are not as obvious as the fist of an abusive boyfriend. The state finally allows a certain set of privileges tied to the marriage of queer couples, but often only to those who most closely mimic the heterosexual two-parent family (and queer couples fought very hard to gain even those few privileges). While smiling gay and lesbian couples celebrate their brand-new marriages on the news in what is unquestionably a monumental and iconic moment for our culture—queer people are still labeled as deviants. Homophobia and lesbophobia (not as defined by transexclusionary radical feminists [TERFs], but actual discrimination against lesbians) still abound and biphobia runs even deeper. Hatred of trans people leads to violent discrimination against them in their quest for even the most basic human rights. And non-white queer people are generally ignored by mainstream organizations, politics, and the media, leaving them for the most part unshielded from even greater violence and discrimination than that which is faced by white queer folks.

---

10 Eisner, *Bi*, 334.
11 Eisner, *Bi*, 231.

For the sake of the most vulnerable in our community and those who will never be protected by the state, we must resist patriarchal coercion to distinguish between "good queers" and "bad queers." Such baseless, nonsensical intra-policing only bolsters cishet dominance; it does nothing to further liberation and in the end hurts all of us. In every oppressed class, we find a few members who are willing to throw their fellows under the bus to gain the applause and rewards offered to them by the dominant class. We see politicians of color supporting racist policies under the illogical guise of respectability. We see women claiming that submission to one's husband is the pinnacle of happiness and fulfillment for all women. We see workers who believe wholeheartedly in the wisdom of Wall Street. In groups as diverse as the queer community, we shouldn't be surprised upon seeing that those queer folk who are already privileged on several axes are accepting entry into the dominant class while decrying the majority of queer people as embarrassing and socially deviant perverts, or simply hushing up the fact that anyone other than khaki-clad, cis male gay couples exist at all.

So, in our identity and our realization of the law's limits, we begin to revolutionize the entire concept of family, bringing it into alignment with the many ways families can be structured. It becomes clear, if we sit and think for even a moment, that the two-parent nuclear family (complete with faithful pet dog and picket fence) is simply not an accurate reflection of many people's realities. By disrupting expectations and artificial requirements, we create space in which families can thrive as they *are*, not as they "should be." Social relationships not constructed along typical family lines, which may nonetheless offer many of the support structures that are associated with family, are given greater respect and weight. We begin to think in ways that will not only benefit us as individuals, but will benefit extended family units, groups in communal living situations, single-parent households, and polyamorous families. By tearing down the privileges afforded to the monogamous, two-parent family unit, we do not devalue the family, nor do we pass judgment on those who choose such a family unit. Rather we elevate human connections, chosen partnerships, and networks of alliance and resistance against patriarchy, capitalism, and white supremacist violence, while allowing for the fluidity of life journeys.

We may well begin to wonder, why should state and corporate interests dictate interpersonal relationships at all? It is obviously inappropriate for an authoritarian, exploitative structure to tell us who we must love, how we must associate ourselves, and under what conditions we should or should not have children. Yet capitalist patriarchy is extremely invested in convincing us that the "cis man + cis woman + good job + children" narrative is ideal for every single person—when in fact, forcing everyone into a single type of family unit is only good for capitalism.

As Gayge Operaista writes in "Radical Queers and Class Struggle: A Match to Be Made":

> We need to oppose the institution of state-sanctioned marriage because it strengthens the nuclear family as the consumptive and reproductive unit of capitalism. . . . Trying to invert the relationship hierarchy to shame people who are happy with a long-term relationship and shared household with a partner does not bring us a step closer to ending capitalism, and ending oppression.[12]

When the intergenerational immigrant family unit is allowed the same status and protection as the white, suburban, two-parent two-children family unit, and when persons of any relationship status are allowed healthcare, access to necessary resources, end-of-life planning, and social respect, everyone will be better off. Such disruption of the privileged, state-approved family unit is bad for hegemonic, consumer-driven state interest, but it is good for real people—for families of all types, for those in communal living situations, for children being raised by those other than their biological parents, for queer folks seeking to establish families of their own. We return to the earlier goals of the queer movement, as described by John D'Emilio in "The Marriage Fight Is Setting Us Back":

> In the 1980s and early 1990s, imaginative queer activists invented such things as 'domestic partnership' and 'second-parent adoption' as ways of recognizing the plethora of family

---

12 Gayge Operaista, "Radical Queers and Class Struggle: A Match to Be Made," in *Queering Anarchism, Addressing and Understanding Power and Desire*, ed. C. B. Daring et al (Oakland, CA: AK Press, 2012), 91.

arrangements that exist throughout the United States. AIDS activists pressed for such things as universal health insurance that would have decoupled perhaps the most significant benefit that marriage offers.[13]

Furthermore, at this crucial point in global history, a creative sharing of resources (resulting from a reimagining and restructuring of family, social, and sexual relationships) could drastically reduce wealth disparity, alleviate poverty, and reduce consumption to a degree that might slow the destruction of the earth. What is good for power structures is not what's good for the people. The subversiveness of bisexual and other non-monosexual identity leads directly to the undermining of multi-faceted oppression as it intersects in that most intimate of relationships: the family.

---

13   John D'Emilio, "The Marriage Fight is Setting Us Back," in *Against Equality: Queer Revolution Not Mere Inclusion,* ed. Ryan Conrad (Oakland, CA: AK Press, 2014), 55–56.

A PERSONAL LOOK AT BISEXUALITY

"Gender and gender identity, sex and sexuality, are spheres of self-discovery that overlap and relate but are not one and the same. . . . There is no formula when it comes to gender and sexuality. . . . I wish that instead of investing in these hierarchies . . . and ranking people according to these rigid standards that ignore diversity in our genders and sexualities, we gave people the freedom and resources to define, determine, and declare who they are."

— Janet Mock[1]

IN OUR IDENTITY, WE SEE THE POSSIBILITY OF SUBVERTING cultural norms surrounding sex, gender, and relationships. Often we first discover this disruption within ourselves. In discovering and owning up to our sexuality, our own deeply-ingrained beliefs are challenged.

If we commit ourselves to resistance, to difference, to queerness, to combating the temptation to assimilation, we find that exploration of our sexuality can change us, strengthen our character, open up new possibilities, and teach us new ways of thinking. We may struggle with decisions regarding lifestyle, passing as straight or gay, and coming out, but by coming out at least to ourselves, we open up the door for change. Changing minds, internal

---

1   Janet Mock, *Redefining Realness: My Path to Womanhood, Identity, Love & So Much More* (New York, NY: Atria Books, 2014), 50.

beliefs, and narratives is a critical component of the move toward a just and equitable society. And the first minds we have to change are our own.

Most of the people included in this collection have written about having to overcome obstacles in order to accept their sexuality. Some were raised in religious homes and had to confront very conservative notions about sexuality and gender roles to even get to a point where self-definition was possible. Others had to break down the monosexist and binary assumptions built into mainstream culture. Many of us did not grow up knowing that non-monosexuality was even a possibility. Many of us were also very isolated from even the mainstream LGBT movement when we were growing up. This isolation is very common for queer young people, and it stems from several factors.

Most American families, especially those raising children a decade or more ago, either did not teach their children about the existence of queer people or did not permit positive narratives about queerness. Decades after the LGBT movement burst into public consciousness, after the Stonewall riots in New York City, after the AIDS crisis, millions of children still grow up not really knowing or understanding the presence of queerness, or that there exists a whole history and movement. Personal identity, including the very words later learned and used in describing individual sexuality and gender, is barely allowed to be a part of a child's consciousness at all. In the last ten years or so, social media and other internet resources have reduced this isolation and knowledge gap, but there are still children who grow up without the knowledge that who they are is okay, and that others like them exist.

The gay movement itself is rigorously policed in the media and the public eye. Only the most assimilationist elements are presented as positive, and even those are often wildly controversial. (The legalization of same-sex marriage has reached an apparent tipping point, where media coverage of the LGBT movement is markedly more positive than it was even five years ago—however, LGBT rights are still regarded as a third rail issue.) The existence of radical, grassroots community is never mentioned. The suggestion that queer people of color exist, or that queer people are advocates for important social causes unrelated to marriage, is totally erased by the mainstream. Each person discovering their own identity has to do a lot of work to realize that there is indeed a place for them in the larger queer community. Queerness is not just for an elite class of gay white men, no matter what the media would have us believe.

Even for the very culturally literate among us, it is difficult to find bisexual role models who might assure us that our identities are real, that we're not alone or crazy. Having to dig through such intentional, unceasing, sometimes even malicious erasure is hard work—and we shouldn't have to engage in hard work or undergo the emotional toll of combatting erasure just to find role models with whom we can identify.

In an atomized society, where class consciousness and solidarity have been suppressed and community has been fragmented into consumer units, where public spaces have been replaced by shopping malls, the discovery of a self that is not branded, that is not prepackaged, and does not fit into the provided mold, can be extremely difficult. The discovery or formation of a community to help in this process is nothing short of radical. From day one, queer people are told there is no place for us in society; we are actively prevented from finding our own community. With increasing gentrification and commercialization of what gayness is allowed to be in the mainstream, poor kids and kids of color learn that not only is queerness not for them, but it is also yet another face of the oppressor. Mainstream erasure of diversity within the queer movement keeps the movement safe and sanitary, while isolating those who need and are capable of creating a radical, authentic, diverse community.

For young queer people coming out in, and coming out of, a rigidly cishet world, education is key. When I say "education," I do not mean an elitist or controlled curriculum; I mean the kind of learning that expands horizons and teaches us things about ourselves and about others that we did not have any way of knowing before. Our culture is still so confused about anything other than standard, approved gender and sexuality, and because of this confusion, many young people coming into the queer community need to learn very basic things. We who already inhabit in this community must provide safe spaces for them to learn; we must know the importance of gentle, forgiving, compassionate education rather than an intimidating pile-on of browbeating, which so frequently happens online when someone missteps. The pile-on is understandable given the abuse faced by queer people every day, but those who are merely uninformed and wish to learn ought to be met with love, rather than rejection.

A Personal Look At Bisexuality

A story might be illustrative here. Growing up in the 1990s in an extremely insular Christian culture, I obtained so few scraps of knowledge about sexuality and gender that I elided several concepts together in my head. When I learned that someone I knew was gay, I became concerned that perhaps I should refer to him with female pronouns. Of course, this was incredibly, laughably incorrect, but in my mind, given only the information I had, it made sense. Although I had been taught that any variance in gender or sexuality was a sin against God, I genuinely wanted to get it right; even if I thought his identity wasn't what God wanted, I didn't want to hurt him by using the wrong pronouns. I listened very carefully to how other people addressed my acquaintance and finally figured out that sexuality and gender identity were not the same thing. Perhaps now, with two more decades of very gradual and incomplete mainstream cultural education on the topic, a young person coming out and into queer culture wouldn't make such a basic mistake. But this personal scenario demonstrates how a very uninformed person can make an honest mistake with nothing but the best of intentions, and how such people are usually the very ones who are also willing to learn and do better.

In exploring our own sexuality, we often encounter questions about gender as well. Even if we do not question our own gender, we might begin to wonder, what does gender mean in the context of sexuality? How do I know for certain what genders I am attracted to?

And often, those of us who had not previously thought deeply about our own gender might begin to question whether we are in fact cisgender. Maybe we are and maybe we aren't; the process of questioning does not assume a foregone conclusion. Whatever the end result, we certainly learn something about ourselves, others, and our sexuality when we begin to think more deeply about gender. In doing so, those of us who are cisgender learn to ally ourselves with trans people, the other daring binary-smashers and border-crossers.

The fact that gender is a construct does not mean it isn't real and doesn't affect our physical existence. Instead, the social construction of gender establishes the source of gender reality in the realm of ideas rather than in the realm of biology. If gender is constructed, it can be deconstructed and reconstructed. Consequently, gender as construct puts the tools of change, of resistance to binaries and cissexism, into our hands. Biological determinism is a fatalistic notion, wherein one's genitals determine an essential part of one's self; this theory is not only clearly false, but also violently erases anyone who identifies as any gender other than that which they were assigned at birth (based on binary assumptions about genital configuration), including trans, genderqueer, and intersex people. Gender as a construct reveals that the power to determine our identities, and the structure of the society we live in, lies with self-actualized individuals working as a community.

If gender can be deconstructed and reconstructed, the same can be done with the meaning assigned to sexuality. When we claim a non-normative identity, we decide that our sexuality is for us—not for somebody else's use or definition. Our ways of loving, and of having sex, do not have to serve patriarchy or capitalism. Of course, living in the society that we do, we find we cannot fully untangle ourselves from oppressive structures that seek to destroy us, whether patriarchy, monosexism, or capitalism, But simultaneously we begin to see our sexuality as a site of freedom, a possibility for resistance, a beginning point of change. By struggling against the "consume and be consumed" roles of heterosexuality as modeled after capitalism, and by declaring that our sexual identity is our *own*, to use for our own good and personal pleasure rather than as a means of reproducing oppression, we strike at the very core of the dehumanizing and alienating capitalist, statist order that seeks to divide us from ourselves.

Much of the initial exploration of sexuality is very personal; it is something one walks through alone, with the help of a few friends, or with the aid of the blessed anonymity the internet provides. Coming out publicly can be an emotionally fraught event for any non-straight and/or non-cis person. Many people, in telling their stories, have a "before" and an "after." Many others come out to countless people in their lives, while remaining closeted to others (I myself am out and very open about my sexuality with most people in my life, but I do not anticipate coming out to my parents at any point). There is no one right way to come out, no one right story to have.

When I was collecting submissions for this book, someone sent me an almost belligerent email asking whether I only wanted stories of oppression. This person seemed to be offended at a suggestion that they felt I was somehow making: that non-monosexuality inevitably means suffering. Of course, this is not the case. There is struggle, there are difficulties, there is oppression, but as many of the people who have written for this book articulate, there is also a great deal of freedom and possibility. Discovering one's own non-normative sexuality is often a transformative, empowering experience. Frequently, I have heard people from across the entire board of queer gender and sexuality express that if given the choice, they would still choose to be queer. The difficulties that can at times overwhelm us do not stem from our own identities—they originate in the cishet, patriarchal world. Queer sexuality and gender are not inherently beset by problems. Thus, when full liberation is achieved, our identities will remain, no longer functioning as sites of struggle and pain.

Discovering who we are is a journey in itself. We may feel compelled to undertake this journey, unable to live any longer as an apparently heterosexual person. We may go through different stages, phases, or fluid spaces before settling into an identity that fits, or we may never settle down to be just one thing—even if that just one thing is the multiplicity contained within bisexuality. The jourhey away from heterosexuality (which is sometimes also bound up in the journey away from the gender one was assigned at birth) does not have to have a fixed destination. We may find that the process of *becoming* continues for our entire lives. That process, however long or short it may be, can create in us a stronger character, a more well-defined self than we would have possessed if we simply remained stagnant, taking our sexuality for granted, or of taking a label for ourselves and leaving it at that.

The mainstream gay movement encourages people to come out. We cannot deny that the great number of publicly-out LGBTQ people have been instrumental in shifting public opinion toward greater approval of non-normative sexuality and gender. However, an individual's decision to come out cannot allow "the good of the movement" to override personal safety concerns. Visibility is important, especially for people so persistently and aggressively erased as non-monosexuals are, but it is not a goal for which anyone should feel compelled to sacrifice their own safety.

In the end, coming out will always be a very personal decision. It can be a moment of both increased visibility and increased difficulty, as some people may face rejection from family members, physical harm at the hand of a partner, loss of a job or housing, and so on. But it can also be a moment of great celebration and freedom—the kind of freedom that can only come by being fully oneself. It can be a desire that becomes so urgent that one feels the obligation to come out regardless of the consequences, or it can be something which one holds close to the chest, disclosing to only a select handful of people throughout one's entire life. And one can be more or less out depending on life circumstances. Any choice an individual makes with regard to coming out is a personal choice, which must be weighed and decided by and for themselves. Such a choice is deeply rooted in personal circumstance and experience, which are things only the individual can know.

Someday, we will create a world in which it is safe to come out, or perhaps a world in which coming out is not even necessary. When such a world exists, it may follow that other, more revolutionary steps are also safer. In today's world, where our very identity brings complication and threats, we may be tempted to lie low. If I myself am vulnerable in one way (or, often in more than one way) simply because of who I am, why would I risk my safety in ways that are avoidable?

But there is risk in safety as well—the risk of excessively personal investment in structures of stability. Although we work for a future where our sexuality does not endanger us, we must simultaneously seize the opportunities presented to us now. Possessing a risky identity can be a radicalizing force in our lives. Enduring a risk that never really goes away can galvanize our courage to take on greater risks. Thus, the power of coming out in a hostile world should not be underestimated. When we are visible and vocal, and work to form a safe community for those who come out, or are considering coming out, we make clear that coming out can be a doorway to greater things. Visibility is a good place to start, but it is only the first step; the discovery of one's identity and the process of coming out is just the beginning.

BISEXUALITY IN THE "LGBT" COMMUNITY

"[U]nderstanding sexuality and gender in terms of rigid, easily identifiable, and heavily policed identities effectively invisibilizes and robs people who do not fit neatly into our available identity categories of a viable social existence."
— C. B. Daring, J. Rogue, Abbey Volcano, and Deric Shannon.[1]

IN DOING RESEARCH FOR THIS PROJECT, I found few books that were fully inclusive of bisexuals, compared to the large number of books available in lesbian and gay literature. Even in the rare (and almost entirely very recently written) works that are inclusive of transgender people, bisexuals remain overlooked (though it is worth noting that books specifically about bisexuals tend to be more inclusive of trans people than LGBT literature at large). Of all the generally LGBT-friendly books I read, the only one that was explicitly inclusive of non-monosexual identities was a rather fluffy, self-help-style book whose stated purpose was "to help make it more likely that people with LGBTQ identities have positive feelings about themselves and experience positive interactions with others."[2] Hardly the tumultuous rainbow of the

---

1   C. B. Daring et al., "Queer Meet Anarchism, Anarchism Meet Queer," in *Queering Anarchism: Addressing and Understanding Power and Desire*, ed. C. B. Daring et al. (Oakland, CA: AK Press, 2012), 12.
2   Ellen D. B. Riggle and Sharon S. Rostosky, *A Positive View of LGBTQ: Embracing*

far left, which we have a right to think would welcome us with open arms. Explicitly leftist books that I read frequently avoided ever saying the word "bisexual," except when spelling out the meaning of the LGBT initialism. For self-avowed "radical" or "progressive" people who claim to write about LGBT issues, collapsing the B into the L and the G with no word of explanation is incredibly irresponsible.

Where the far-left queer movement might be somewhat lacking in terminology, specific information, and resources for bisexual and other non-monosexual people, the deficits of the mainstream LGBT movement can be outright harmful. Mainstream movements are so very often focused exclusively on gays and lesbians (with the smiling, young, white, and upper-class gay male couple as the archetype) that some writers who are more sensitive to the broad spectrum of queerness do not even refer to these movements as LGBT. Shiri Eisner refers to the "GGGG movement" (for gay, gay, gay, gay), and the editors of *Queering Anarchism* write it as "G(lbt)."

It is not simply a problem of the erasure, the focus of mainstream gay movements on only a certain type of gay person, or the overt biphobia. Mainstream LGBT movements also materially benefit from bi erasure. As documented by the San Francisco Human Rights Commission in 2011, most studies on the needs of queer communities collapse the bisexual population into the lesbian and gay population, thereby inflating the recorded instances of suicide, domestic violence, and drug use among gays and lesbians.[3] The San Francisco Human Rights Commission describes the results of such flawed research: "It may . . . result in interventions not reaching or not being effective for key populations. . . . This means that even though bisexuals may have greater need, the resources primarily end up benefiting lesbians and gay men."[4] Even when "the word 'bisexual' shows up in an organization's name or mission statement," the organization often "doesn't offer programming that addresses the specific needs of bisexuals."[5] This is not to say that such material benefits to gays and lesbians, at the expense of bisexuals, happen through any malice or specific plots to disenfranchise

---

Identity and Cultivating Well-Being (Lanham, MD: Rowman & Littlefield, 2012), 2.

3 Also see similar effects reported in Kaestle and Ivory, "A Forgotten Sexuality."
4   San Francisco Human Rights Commission, "Bisexual Invisibility," 13.
5   San Francisco Human Rights Commission, "Bisexual Invisibility," 5.

certain sexual minorities. It is simply the natural outcome of biphobia, bi erasure, and constant striving by the mainstream gay movement to pander to the most centrist elements of society and media.

Not only is the material distribution of resources and attention hostile to non-monosexual people in LGBT spaces, many common catchphrases and nuggets of conventional wisdom that are bandied about often exclude our experiences, making us feel yet again that we do not quite fit in.

In order to gain greater acceptance from the heterosexual world, proponents of gay rights and gay marriage cultivate a "born this way" narrative. But such a narrative is not as helpful as it may appear to be. Although straight folks may find comfort in believing that we just can't help it, saying we were "born this way" places us in a defensive posture rather than a celebratory one. In addition, if straight folks are only compelled to accept an amount of queerness that "cannot be helped," then they are not compelled to accept bisexuals who aren't willing to pass as straight. Furthermore, the "born this way" narrative can create a great deal of confusion or alienation for those whose sexuality has evolved and may still be evolving, those whose sexuality is fluid, and those who have never felt a fixed sort of destiny about their sexuality. In the end, bisexuals and non-monosexuals as a whole are not creating a revolution for who and what we were born as—we are creating a revolution for who and what we are now, and who we will become. We are creating a revolution where our personhood, in all its aspects, can evolve without fear and without being forced into oppressive boxes and narratives that are not our own.

In a manner closely related to the "born the way" narrative, the complete rejection of language of choice among the mainstream gay community often leads to rejection and marking of bisexuals as "not really queer." After all, we can *choose* to pass as straight. The assumption, of course, is a troubling one: who would be queer if they could choose not to be? It casts bisexuals as tourists, as imposters, as people who are experimenting but will eventually go back to a safe, heterosexual lifestyle; it asserts that while we may not have chosen to be bisexual, we do seem to have a choice as to what kind of partnerships we might enter into, and in doing so avoid the persecution of being truly queer. But when we defend ourselves against accusations of not being queer enough (which, in truth, usually translates to not being out enough or oppressed enough), we end up participating in an unhelpful "oppression olympics" whereby we must prove our identity by how greatly we've suffered. Suffice it to say, regardless of whether or not we appear to live a heteronormative or homonormative lifestyle (and who can really choose the person they are attracted to, or with whom they fall in love?), we are *still queer enough*. Even a person who identifies as bisexual now but later identifies as straight, in the moments when they identify as bisexual, they are queer enough.

What is especially troubling about the mainstream gay movement is its eagerness, and almost single-minded focus, on gaining access to institutions of privilege and power.[6] This alone is enough to alienate many progressive and leftist queer folk from the mainstream movement. Would it really be a great advance if, for example, there were an openly bisexual general in the United States military? Does a non-monosexual person in a position of power make the world a better place if that power is used to invade other countries and advance imperialist and capitalist concerns? How is the movement at all benefited when such actions would likely be to the detriment of ordinary queer or LGBT people in the invaded and occupied territories?

Even when LGBT people are in positions of power or privilege in less harmful institutions, it is important to question why this goal seems to constitute the entirety of the movement agenda. Is it an attempt at trickle-down liberation? History has taught us that trickle-down liberation does not work nearly as well as we might hope, particularly given the allotment of time and resources invested in the attempt. Most often, when certain members of a marginalized group gain access to truly privileged positions of institutional power, they adopt the values and interests of those institutions, instead of advancing the interests and values of the marginalized group whence they came. We see this discrepancy occur, for example, when politicians of color rush to urge nonviolent Black protesters to be "peaceful" in their response to white supremacist violence, as though the Black community is the problem. We see it in commonplace, apparently innocuous situations, like when a CEO claims to care about the environment; instead of exploring deep ecological alternatives to the exploitative destruction of the earth, they turn "green" into a brand and actually increase consumption of resources through

---

6 A thorough critique of this tendency of the mainstream gay movement is found in Ryan Conrad, ed. *Against Equality: Queer Revolution Not Mere Inclusion* (Oakland, CA: AK Press, 2014).

their "green"-branded products. When radical or progressive movements are so assimilated and packaged, it has a deeply demoralizing effect on the remainder of the movement. When those who we are taught to look up to are hand in hand with oppressors who preach acquiescence, assimilation, and respectability, we have achieved only the commercialization of our most important values.

Even when a person from a marginalized community or movement maintains their integrity upon gaining power within the existing system, no single achievement is the sole vehicle of liberation. The more sequestered an accomplishment is in largely inaccessible, elite institutions, the less likely it is to benefit the ordinary queer person, or advance the cause of liberation. More than any other position of privilege, the academic role is likely to contribute to the greater movement, through teaching, changing research methodology, and exploring queer theory. If we are to remake ideas and learn new methods of action and existence, theoretical discussions and vocabulary expansion are essential parts of that process. Finding a word that describes one's reality with a level of accuracy that no other word has yet attained is a marvelous experience and allows for greater clarity of thought and action. That's a good thing, indeed!

However, locating a possible source of liberation within the academic sphere is problematic, due to issues of access and hierarchy that plague academic institutions. Luckily, popular social media platforms such as Twitter and Tumblr have become locations for ordinary people to take words and concepts once locked up in ivory towers and cultivate them in everyday life. The evolution of consciousness and of action made possible by popularizing aspects of queer theory cannot be discredited. By essentially crowdsourcing queer theory, social media platforms and blogging communities allow activists and others with real-life experience and vital stakes in queer issues to advance ideas by leaps and bounds, and then turn those ideas into concrete action. It may be that even now (and if not now, sometime in the near future), ordinary people will outpace academics in their development of ideas and consciousness surrounding queer liberation.

So long as theory remains located in institutions of power, its ability to affect mass social changes is vastly decreased. When put into the hands of the people, theory is wedded to action, and real difference can be made in society. When people discuss ideas and put undistorted terminology to use in their everyday life, it becomes impossible to keep those ideas in discrete boxes. Many social media users regularly discuss queer theory alongside feminism and race; all of the theory is applied to everyday actions and interactions, and constantly evolves through interaction with other social media users. It's a powerful method that could not easily be replicated by an academic paper.

The more egalitarian, bottom-up, and margins-inward a movement is, the better. However, for the past few decades, the mainstream gay movement has proved itself to be none of those things. As Sarah Schulman documents in *The Gentrification of the Mind*, the "heart of gay liberation" was once "a melding of the human need for free sexual expression [and] a sense of social justice,"[7] but after the AIDS crisis the gay movement became steadily more and more "gentrified"—that is, invested in privilege rather than community, revolution, authenticity, justice, and truth. For those who understand the deeper revolutionary potential of queerness, such a shift can seem like nothing less than sabotage. Those who were already in privileged positions neutered the movement and consolidated the remains for themselves, while the mainstream world swooped in to assimilate it at the very moment gay people were at their most vulnerable. Bisexuals, pansexuals, and other non-monosexuals are casualties of this gentrification, both metaphorically and literally (e.g. the brutal police discrimination against queer young people, especially those of color, on the streets of gentrified neighborhoods. As non-monosexuals, we have the potential to disrupt the respectability in which the mainstream gay movement is so deeply entrenched. Consequently, we are not welcomed into either that movement's ideological or physical space.

Rather than withdrawing from the queer community at large, or individually scrambling to access power and privilege for ourselves at the expense of the less privileged members of the community, we need to learn from the difficulties we face at the hands of the mainstream gay movement— just as much as we learn from the oppression wreaked upon us by cishet patriarchy. Using what we have learned from and about the spurious binary of monosexuality and the communities invested in that binary, we can create our own unique community that will strive toward a better future for all.

---

[7] Sarah Schulman, *The Gentrification of the Mind* (Berkeley, CA: University of California Press, 2012), 161.

THE BISEXUAL COMMUNITY, ALLYSHIP, ACTIVISM, AND REVOLUTIONARY POTENTIAL

"Bisexual movements need to remember their own power—not apologize for who they are or try to fit into constrictive notions of normalcy, but to stand up for their identities and the threat to normalcy that comes along with them: fighting for liberation rather than privilege, for the destruction of the system rather than a place at the table, for the revolution rather than for rights."

— Shiri Eisner[1]

ALTHOUGH THERE HAS BEEN NO DISCRETE CATEGORY OF BISEXUALITY until the 20th century, we find that throughout history, family and kinship networks, sexuality, and erotic partnerships have always been more complex and varied than the dominant narrative would permit. Up until the late 19th century, sexual behavior was not organized into distinct, medicalized identity categories.[2] People from all walks of life, whether political radicals or respectable members of society, engaged in sexual activity with people of all genders. Most of our ancestors—and most people from any other

---

1   Eisner, *Bi*, 316.
2   For further discussion of this point, see: Eisner, *Bi*, 14–20; Lachlan MacDowall, "Historicizing Contemporary Bisexuality," *Journal of Bisexuality* 9:1 (2009): 3–15, accessed July 20, 2014, doi: 10.1080/15299710802659989.

culture in the world—would be confused by the current monosexist cultural assumption that any homosexual or homoerotic behavior must necessarily confines one to a single category of sexuality.[3] During many historical periods, homoeroticism (if not actual sexual contact) between people otherwise assumed to be heterosexual (anachronistic as the application of that term is, in this case), was considered normal and healthy. The bi community today is historically unique only in the clarity of our self-identification. People like us have not enjoyed the same sanctioned, privileged position as heterosexuals have, but we have not always been quite as oppressed and marginalized as a surface reading of history would suggest.

Although we enjoy greater clarity of self-identification than those like us may have enjoyed in the past, it is still almost impossible to point to a discrete entity and call it "the bisexual community." Compared to other sexual minorities, we have few, if any, brick-and-mortar institutions that are our own, few organizations that are just for us, few programs, few research papers, few books.[4] As much as I might wish we all could have weekly meetings where we could eat cookies and plan out how to smash the white supremacist, cishet patriarchy, we don't—though it would be such fun to see the right-wing news media flip out over these meetings! For the most part we have to organize community online or within our existing circle of friends.

As we begin to build community around a shared sexual nonconformity, there arises the immediate temptation of assimilation and respectability, which we need to reject before it even gets a foot in the door. If divisive ploys of hierarchy and power are built into our foundation, they will be that much harder to remove once the problems they inevitably create become urgent.

We must also avoid the temptation to distinguish between "good" and "bad" bisexuals. Although it might be easy to simply reject the stereotypes used to dismiss us, we must instead, as Eisner discusses in detail,[5] reject the underlying insinuations that give those stereotypes power. For instance, instead of denying that some bisexuals may be promiscuous, we need to reject

---

3   See, for instance, Sharon Marcus, *Between Women: Friendship, Desire, and Marriage in Victorian England* (Princeton, NJ: Princeton University Press, 2007) for a discussion of female same-sex relationships of a wide variety in Victorian England, or for a general discussion of cultural and historical views of sexuality, see Burleson, *Bi America*, 29–37.

4   See Burleson, *Bi America*, 62–64.

5   Eisner, *Bi*, 35–49.

the unspoken implication that promiscuity is inherently bad. If promiscuity is not inherently bad, then it does not matter whether or not some bisexuals are promiscuous; thus, a non-monogamous bisexual is not a bad person. Affirming that ethical non-monogamy is a valid expression of sexuality, and by that definition has a place within the non-monosexual community, ought to be more important to us than attempting to appear respectable by the standards of people who condemn non-monogamy.

Just as we take care to not divide "good" and "bad" bisexuals, we also must avoid sorting people into "good" and "bad" categories based on their perceived level of radicalness or commitment to "the cause." To illustrate, the practical commitments involved in parenting young children might leave a parent with less time and energy to devote to an organization or movement, and they may be more likely to choose stability over a precarious, ideals-driven life. Some people are faced with health challenges or mental illness (and in fact, bisexuals face higher rates of mental illness than other sexual minorities do),[6] which can make even performing even simple daily tasks like brushing one's teeth an enormous accomplishment. Of course, not everyone must think the same way about everything, or live their lives in exactly the way that *you* choose to live your life. By extracting ourselves from mono-narratives surrounding sexuality, we can become open and compassionate to differences and degrees of nonconformity in other areas of life as well, expanding our willingness for diverse, multi-faceted community. Constantly policed boundaries help no one; indeed, diverse viewpoints, abilities, and interests, united around the shared purpose of fighting oppression, are a strength. Getting away from the fear of being a "bad radical" and refraining from judging others for being "too extreme" or not extreme enough allows for compassion, self-care, and a strong community less prone to burnout.

Another challenge we face at the very outset of defining the parameters of a non-monosexual community is sustaining acknowledgment and acceptance of sexual fluidity without erasing bisexuality, pansexuality, and other more fixed non-monosexual identities. Often, we defend against common misperceptions, that subtlety can be easily lost. We can be so busy fighting assumptions that we're "just experimenting," "going through a

---

6   San Francisco Human Rights Commission, LGBT Advisory Committee. "Bisexual Invisibility: Impacts and Recommendations." San Francisco, CA, 2011. 12–14.

phase," or "in denial about being gay," that we fail to create a safe space for individuals whose identity is fluid. As those of us with fairly fixed identities (which are expansive in their own right) affirm the reality and validity of our identities, we must simultaneously work to change the understanding of boundaries and categories in order to allow fluid sexual identities to also be accepted as real and valid. Not everyone who has had sex with people of more than one gender in the past identifies as bisexual now; some people move through a period of identifying as bisexual as they shift from heterosexual to homosexual attraction. Even as those of us with a more fixed identity do not want our stories erased, we must take care to not unwittingly erase the stories of those with fluid identities, either.

For we must all stand together—we are the misfits of the misfits, the ones who don't belong, even in a community of those who don't fit into mainstream culture. We have a choice: We can seek to make ourselves belong by throwing others under the bus for being too slutty, too queer, too far outside the lines. We can bow to the pressure from the cishet world and from the mainstream gay community to mold ourselves into something acceptable. Or we can proudly be something *other*. We can be people who accept the outcasts, people who create a safe space in the queer community for all non-monosexuals and for those who are just passing through. We can be people who seek to create safety in other places we inhabit, for the benefit of other misfits who might not have a sexuality similar to our own. We can allow our thinking to be colonized, our actions to be exclusionary, and our identities to be assimilated to the demands of the dominant social order—or we can use our misfit status to break open borders and smash barriers. We can create strength from our uniqueness, instead of tidying it up to make a pleasing aesthetic for people who find us abhorrent. The process of changing social narratives around sexuality will take patience, but in the meantime, it's necessary for us, as the "middle of the rainbow," to create these safe spaces for our peers who do not fit into a simple, one-word explanation of sexuality.

Why should we be stingy with our identity at all? It's not as though there's only so much queerness to go around. Why function under capitalist logic, fearing scarcity and inadequacy? If someone wants to explore the possibility of bisexuality, if they call themselves bisexual for a short period of time, or if they pass through as part of a transitional phase before identifying as gay or lesbian, why shouldn't we be happy to party with them while they're here? Even people who are only able to express bisexual desire when under the influence of alcohol or drugs should be welcomed when they choose to show up; their repression is the fault of a violently heterosexist society. Taking our frustration at that society out on others who are oppressed by its deluded ideals does nothing but divide us from potential friends, partners, and allies. Let's be hospitable, because being exclusionary and judgemental, policing our borders, and getting hung up on who's *really* bisexual, is only reenacting the power dynamics of capitalist patriarchy. That's something we specifically do not want to mimic.

As non-monosexuals, we have experienced first-hand the harm of a binary narrative and thus we know clearly that must never fall into the trap of creating another such narrative. We must reject the notion that permanence is required for desire to have validity, for it is unfair to cultivate any artificial standard to which we hold ourselves or others. Telling our personal stories is not meant to create a single correct narrative to which all others must conform—it is a practice by which diverse experiences can be entered into a dialogue that results in action, theory, and movement building. Insist on the reality and validity of your own journey, and believe in the reality and validity of others' journeys as well, for in these individual stories, across which many themes may be repeated, we learn what oppressions may face us, and we gain insights for revolution.

We tell our stories to each other but as we move forward, it is of great importance that we also tell them to those outside of our community. As we say "We are here, just as we are, not as you want us to be," we audibly resist assimilation. As much as possible, we should tell the truth about ourselves. That is the first step toward disrupting the cishet structures surrounding us.

In one of the essays in this collection, Kierstyn King, bisexual and non-binary, writes, "My existence seems to break people's brains." It's an unfortunate fact that when we are honest about ourselves in a hostile, cishet world, we will all to some extent encounter that same reaction. But if we break down people's ideas of what ought to be, and deconstruct the boxes built inside their heads, we may be able to change their minds for the better. "Breaking people's brains" is a small price to pay in the quest for a world where we aren't silenced, abused, raped, and treated as inferior. It is the necessary precursor to building up a more just world for everyone: not only non-monosexuals, but trans and genderqueer people as well.

In the end, I'm not personally worried about causing a little mental distress to straight cis people who have a hard time comprehending bisexuality. I see the pain my peers endure for not fitting into a sexual binary, and I can spare no sympathy for people who want a clearly-defined, simple world at our expense. Our very existence threatens hierarchies that privilege heterosexuals over queers, and while acknowledging and discussing this confrontational existence is painful to close-minded folks, it can be a gasp of recognition and a homecoming for people who didn't even know they were closeted.

We inhabit and pass between dominant cishet cultures and various queer cultures, even in our most intimate relationships. As bisexuals, we are likely to be romantically and/or sexually partnered with one or more people whose sexualities differ from our own. As we participate in these relationships, we confront the ableist, biphobic stoking of fears that bisexuals are "disease vectors." This term is a stand-in, as Eisner points out, for the belief that bisexuals will infect "normal" people with queerness.[7] Eisner explains this misconception by the fact that many bisexuals can pass as straight at some times and in some places: "Passing . . . plays out on hegemonic fears of infiltration and invasion, reflecting dominant groups' fear of not being able to distinguish between 'us' and 'them.' . . . This is a direct threat to the distribution of power and privilege in society."[8]

Although we may not be able to turn a cishet partner queer just by the sheer force of our identity, we can bring change to the cishet world through our friendships and romantic and sexual relationships. To bridge queer and cishet culture, we can share with cishet and monosexual people what we have learned about subversive models of relationships, consent, intimacy, and ways of confronting power hierarchies. Cishet and monosexual people do not have the same experience we do, born as it is out of our unique identity—but they can learn from us.

Bisexual people in relationships with straight people need not allow themselves to be controlled by fears of engulfment by the cishet patriarchy. Instead, we should consciously and intentionally seek to conduct our

---

[7] Eisner, *Bi*, 46–47. For a serious investigation of whether the "disease vector" claim has any basis in reality, see Burleson, *Bi America*, 135–150.
[8] Eisner, *Bi*, 118.

relationships *queerly*, by exploring non-oppressive, liberated models of relating to one another in every area of life. Of course it is never our responsibility to remain with abusive or oppressive partners simply in an attempt to teach them to be better people, but we can look to the fundamentals of our identity to provide resources and support for constructively transforming our healthy relationships, now or in the future.

Those of us who are attracted to people of more than one gender have to think in greater depth and complexity about our relationships. Since our world isn't divided into neat categories of people who are potential partners and people who are not, each relationship must be taken for what it is made up of; the circumstances, personalities, attraction, and emotional intensity that all play a greater role in determining our social, sexual, and romantic relationships more so than gender. (The silly question posed by endless romcoms of whether or not men and women can just be friends holds no weight for us; if we can't be friends with anyone of a gender we might potentially be attracted to, it would be impossible for us to ever have friends.)

In this intentionality and autonomy that we bring to sex and relationships, we have an opportunity to promote the necessity of consent. Our approach to sex and relationships does not necessarily follow a set script, and so with no controlling narrative to make us take each step of the process for granted (whether engaging in a one-night hookup or a long-term relationship), consent is always found to be necessary. Ethical sex, we also find, is not about who or how many people an individual sleeps with. It is about freely given consent between adult people. When all other rules are stripped away, consent remains. Although others may use our sexuality as an excuse to harm us through rape or domestic violence, we have the tremendous power to use our sexuality to create and promote healthy sex lives for ourselves and our partners.

We also tend to find that these boundaries and the necessity of consent play a more explicit role in our lives than in the lives of most monosexuals. Unlike people who engage in homosocial behavior and emotionally intense relationships with those of the same gender, and rest easy in the assurance that "nothing will ever happen" because both parties are straight, bisexuals must negotiate (without the benefit of preconceived notions) the realization that while not all our emotionally intense relationships need to have a sexual component, it is simultaneously possible that any such relationship might become sexual if the circumstances are right and consent is given. This nuanced way of navigating relationships is absolutely something that can be taught to cishet people. We can responsibly destabilize the perpetually heteronormative reading of emotionally intense same-sex relationships, and we can destabilize the continual hypersexualization of emotionally intense queer relationships and between cishet people of different genders.

We live in a society totally centered on narratives about love between a cishet man and a cishet woman. As non-monosexuals, we get to question that narrative. We get to open the playing field up to a full array of sexual, erotic, romantic, and emotional relationships, and we get to advocate a complex, textured understanding of love. Just as bisexuality and non-monosexuality as a whole opens up the possibility for sexual relationships between people of all genders, so too can it restore other types of love to the narrative of a truly fulfilling human life. Just as we do not have to end up in a life-long, exclusive heterosexual pairing, we also do not have to locate all sexual, romantic, erotic, emotionally intense, loving, and affectionate meaning for our life in a single relationship. Our expansion of the cultural conversation about love beyond the boundaries of romantic cishet relationships, and beyond the boundaries of the picket-fence nuclear family, can only result in a healthy change.

Important movements start small, but even in the limited space we now occupy, we have begun to lay the groundwork for bigger things. As we move forward from laying the groundwork for what our own community will look like, and from transforming interpersonal relationships at the micro-level, we can look at the macro-level world around us and formulate plans for how to change it. During this process, we discover another strength within ourselves. The roots of our oppression are many, each facet containing multiple other aspects, and so our response must also be multiple, diverse, expansive—poly, not mono. As people who fall in the middle or outside of the sexuality spectrum, non-monosexuals (as well as genderqueer, trans, and agender people) are accustomed to crossing boundaries. We've learned that strict categories are not able to define who we are. Binaries have failed us. Mono-narratives fall short. We can take this experience—the constant rejection of the "either/or" narrative that works to misshape our thinking about ourselves—from our own lives, and use it inform how we change and re-shape society. The patterns of thinking that are ever-evolving from our queerness are invaluable. People who are shaped by mono-thinking may see such an approach as scattered or lacking focus, but the multiplicity of our existence and action outside of socially approved boxes is one of our greatest strengths. Oppression of queer people, and oppression faced by people in the queer community on the basis of other factors such as gender or race, stems from many sources: material, ideological, political, and so on. We must become just as accustomed to poly-thinking in our analysis and modes of action as we are accustomed to being attracted to various genders.

We may find that, while we share the non-monosexual identity umbrella, we are all interested and active in a wide array of political and social issues. Some of us may focus on bisexual issues. Others may focus on gender, economic problems, prison abolition, anti-war or anti-imperialist action. No matter the issue, we must all cultivate an awareness of other realms of justice; truly intersectional activism never places a single issue in a vacuum. This is especially important as we find encounter people in our own community who are affected by diverse challenges, oppressions, and systems of injustice. If we seek true liberation, we cannot limit ourselves to issues that are overtly and immediately related to sexuality.

As a simple thought experiment, choose an area of justice that is related to sexuality, and see how many other political and social justice issues you can connect to it. For instance, bisexuals have unique healthcare needs. So, what about universal healthcare? Or access to healthcare for bisexuals in prison? What about the injustice of our prison-industrial complex as a whole? Can you connect the increased militarization of American police forces? What about violent white supremacy that leads to the death of Black people at the hands of police and white vigilantes? What about the U.S. military's imperialist oppression of non-white people abroad? What about the exploitation of workers in sweatshops owned by United States capitalist interests that are advanced by the military? What about the unsustainability of environmental exploitation? What about justice for immigrants displaced by environmental disasters? What about the sexual assault of undocumented women held in prisons along the US/Mexico border? And on and on it goes; there is no isolated issue. At every link in the chain, we find others in our community who are affected. Just as every person is connected, so too is every political and social justice issue.

As we become more conscious of the erasure we face as bisexuals, we must not lose sight of the structures of oppression that we ourselves participate in and perpetuate. Calling out the wrongdoing or wrong thinking of others is necessary, but we must always practice confrontation of our own wrongdoing and wrong thinking, as well. Even as we seek to tear down structures that oppress us, we must also work to tear down structures that may benefit us but oppress others.

By standing in solidarity with people who are not like us, we are standing in solidarity with each other. Bisexuality, pansexuality, polysexuality, sexual fluidity, and other non-monosexual identities encompass an enormously diverse group of people. So to reach the greatest personal sway and alliance, be visible where you are, and offer support and resources to those standing elsewhere. You may become more aware of the non-monosexual community through encounters with non-monosexual people in your own, seemingly unrelated political or social work, or you may become aware of certain political and social issues through the realization that your fellow non-monosexuals face oppression and are present in every movement for liberation. No matter how such awareness occurs, the bisexual community is in a position to become integral to the fight against the current oppressive world order.

With intentionality, any justice work you do can end up benefitting bisexuals in some way, and education about issues facing bisexual and non-monosexual people in general can increase the effectiveness of your work or expand the possibilities within that space. For example, let's say you are working on a rape prevention campaign at a rape crisis center. Your work benefits bisexuals in a tangible way, as we are one of the populations most likely to face sexual violence. You can bring greater awareness to the particular plight of bisexuals even as you continue to work against rape in totality. You can develop educational materials to help your organization better serve the individual needs of bisexuals, and in the process, you might also challenge your fellow workers to develop similar materials to help serve other particularly at-risk groups, such as trans people or undocumented immigrants. The same sort of approach easily translates to work in domestic violence shelters, mental healthcare facilities, support services for incarcerated populations, and of course political action groups centered on sexuality and gender.

Although we may begin small, with personal reflection on who we love and who we are attracted to, being bisexual has the enormous potential to shape who we are, how we think, and how we take action. We face obstacles and oppression, and we face danger even when we pass in the straight community—it is true. However, we find that when we undertake an intentional journey of honesty, and when we take lessons learned from our identity and apply that first-hand wisdom elsewhere, we gain integrity, strength, and community. Furthermore, we gain the ability to effectively deepen and broaden our impact on the advancement of justice and liberation.

No matter how much I read, think, imagine, and write about revolution, no matter how many uprisings I have seen in recent days, the first image that always comes to my mind is the barricade scene in *Les Miserables*: common folk tearing up the pavement and rationing weapons, facing down soldiers and hoping to last the night. But the reality is that revolution is multi-faceted, a simultaneous confrontation and destruction of the old order and an imagining, creation, and organization of a new order. Sometimes something breaks, and a riot causes a movement to explode across public consciousness. But mostly, revolution goes on in small ways all around us, all the time. The people most prepared to help when larger movements begin, when protestors in the streets face down cops in riot gear, are the ones who are practiced in both destruction and creation.

The suggestions I have made in this reflection about how our sexuality can contribute to social change and revolution are by no means comprehensive. This is a beginning, not an exhaustive how-to manual. I trust that you have far more and much better ideas than I have presented here. If you are busy right now subverting norms and challenging expectations, creating alternative spaces, directing resources toward those in need rather than allowing them to pool up in the hands of the wealthy, you are already practicing revolution in your daily life. We all dream of the day when everything happens all at once and the unjust, oppressive systems of our society are rapidly overthrown, but there's no need to wait for that. Revolution is here and now.

Get started.

BIBLIOGRAPHY

Burleson, William E. *Bi America: Myths, Truths, and Struggles of an Invisible Community.* Binghamton, NY: Harrington Park Press, 2005.

Conrad, Ryan, ed. *Against Equality: Queer Revolution Not Mere Inclusion.* Oakland, CA: AK Press, 2014.

Conrad, Ryan. "Gay Marriage and Queer Love." In *Queering Anarchism: Addressing and Understanding Power and Desire*, edited by C. B. Daring, J. Rogue, Deric Shannon, and Abbey Volcano, 18–22. Oakland, CA: AK Press, 2012. PDF e-book.

Daring, C. B., J. Rogue, Deric Shannon, and Abbey Volcano, Ed. *Queering Anarchism: Addressing and Understanding Power and Desire.* Oakland, CA: AK Press, 2012. PDF e-book.

Daring, C. B., J. Rogue, Abbey Volcano, and Deric Shannon. "Queer Meet Anarchism, Anarchism Meet Queer." In *Queering Anarchism: Addressing and Understanding Power and Desire*, edited by C. B. Daring, J. Rogue, Deric Shannon, and Abbey Volcano, 8–17. Oakland, CA: AK Press, 2012. PDF e-book.

Bibliography

D'Emilio, John. "The Marriage Fight is Setting Us Back." In *Against Equality: Queer Revolution Not Mere Inclusion*, edited by Ryan Conrad, 51–56. Oakland, CA: AK Press, 2014.

Duffy, Owen. "Bisexual Asylum Seeker Facing Imminent Deportation From UK to Jamaica." *The Guardian*, May 5, 2015. Accessed June 20, 2015. www.theguardian.com/uk-news/2015/may/05/bisexual-jamaica-asylum-seeker-facing-imminent-deportation-from-uk

Echols, Alice. *Scars of Sweet Paradise: The Life and Times of Janis Joplin*. New York, NY: Henry Holt and Company, 1999.

Eisner, Shiri. *Bi: Notes for a Bisexual Revolution*. Berkeley, CA: Seal Press, 2013.

Ehrhardt, Michelle. "DC Comics: Harley Quinn & Poison Ivy Are Girlfriends 'Without Monogamy.'" *Out*, June 15, 2015. Accessed June 20, 2015. www.out.com/popnography/2015/6/15/dc-comics-harley-quinn-poison-ivy-are-girlfriends-without-monogamy

Gladstone. "5 Gay Guys Who Got More Women Than Most Straight Men." *Cracked*, April 27, 2012. Accessed June 20, 2015. http://www.cracked.com/blog/5-gay-guys-who-got-more-women-than-most-straight-men

Heckert, Jamie. "Anarchy without Opposition." In *Queering Anarchism: Addressing and Understanding Power and Desire*, edited by C. B. Daring, J. Rogue, Deric Shannon, and Abbey Volcano, 50–59. Oakland, CA: AK Press, 2012. PDF e-book.

Kaestle, Christine Elizabeth, and Adrienne Holz Ivory. "A Forgotten Sexuality: Content Analysis of Bisexuality in the Medical Literature over Two Decades." *Journal of Bisexuality* 12:1 (2012): 35–48. Accessed August 11, 2014. doi: 10.1080/15299716.2012.645701.

Kate and Deeg. "Marriage is Still the Opiate of the Queers." In *Against Equality: Queer Revolution Not Mere Inclusion*, edited by Ryan Conrad, 45-49. Oakland, CA: AK Press, 2014.

MacDowall, Lachlan. "Historicising Contemporary Bisexuality." *Journal of Bisexuality* 9:1 (2009): 3–15. Accessed July 20, 2014. doi: 10.1080/15299710802659989.

Marcus, Sharon. *Between Women: Friendship, Desire, and Marriage in Victorian England*. Princeton, NJ: Princeton University Press, 2007.

Mock, Janet. *Redefining Realness: My Path to Womanhood, Identity, Love & So Much More*. New York, NY: Atria Books, 2014.

Mogul, Joey L., Andrea J. Ritchie, and Kay Whitlock. *Queer (In)Justice: The Criminalization of LGBT People in the United States*. Boston, MA: Beacon Press, 2011.

Operaista, Gayge. "Radical Queers and Class Struggle: A Match to Be Made." In *Queering Anarchism: Addressing and Understanding Power and Desire*, edited by C. B. Daring, J. Rogue, Deric Shannon, and Abbey Volcano, 87–96. Oakland, CA: AK Press, 2012. PDF e-book.

Riggle, Ellen D. B. and Sharon S. Rostosky. *A Positive View of LGBTQ: Embracing Identity and Cultivating Well-Being*. Lanham, MD: Rowman & Littlefield, 2012.

Roberts, Dorothy. *Killing the Black Body: Race, Reproduction, and the Meaning of Liberty*. New York, NY: Vintage Books, 1997.

San Filippo, Maria. *The B Word: Bisexuality in Contemporary Film and Television*. Bloomington, IN: Indiana University Press, 2013.

San Francisco Human Rights Commission, LGBT Advisory Committee. "Bisexual Invisibility: Impacts and Recommendations." San Francisco, CA, 2011

.Schulman, Sarah. *The Gentrification of the Mind*. Berkeley, CA: University of California Press, 2012.

Starhawk. *Dreaming the Dark: Magic, Sex, and Politics*. Boston, MA: Beacon Press, 1997.

Bibliography

Walters, Suzanna Danuta. *The Tolerance Trap: How God, Genes, and Good Intentions Are Sabotaging Gay Equality*. New York, NY: New York University Press, 2014.

Wolf, Sherry. *Sexuality and Socialism: History, Politics, and Theory of LGBT Liberation*. Chicago, IL: Haymarket Books, 2009.

Yoshino, Kenji. "The Epistemic Contract of Bisexual Erasure." *Stanford Law Review* 52 (2000): 353–455.

Young, Rebecca M. and Ilan H. Meyer. "The Trouble with 'MSM' and 'WSW': Erasure of the Sexual-Minority Person in Public Health Discourse." *American Journal of Public Health* 95 (2005): 1144–1149.

Zinn, Howard. *A People's History of the United States: 1492–Present*. New York, NY: Harper Perennial, 2005.

OoOA!

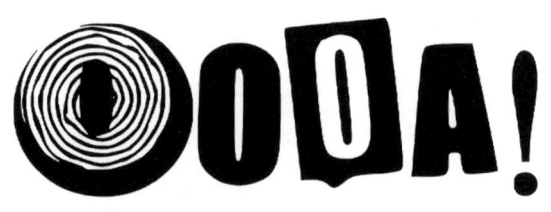

ON OUR OWN AUTHORITY! PUBLISHING
ATLANTA, GEORGIA

On Our Own Authority! Publishing (OooA!) is an autonomous research press in Atlanta, Georgia, founded in 2012. Specializing in anarchist studies and radical literature, we publish social movement history, post-colonial history, and studies of global political thought, emphasizing themes of anti-colonialism, direct democracy, and workers' self-management.

Other titles available from On Our Own Authority!:

Lenni Brenner and Matthew Quest, *Black Liberation and Palestine Solidarity*.

Joseph Edwards, *Workers' Self-Management in the Carribean*.

Emma Goldman and Alexander Berkman, *To Remain Silent Is Impossible*.

Sen Katayama, *The Labor Movement in Japan*.

Eusi Kwayana, *The Bauxite Strike and the Old Politics*.

Louise Michel, William Morris, et al., *The Commune: Paris, 1871*.

Kimathi Mohammed, *Organization and Spontaneity*.

David Weir, *Jean Vigo and the Anarchist Eye*.

Ida B. Wells, *Lynch Law in Georgia & Other Writings*.

Visit us online at www.oooabooks.org